Getting Your
Own Back

To. MRS P. MIDDLETON
99. ROEDALE ROAD
HOLLINGDEAN, BRIGHTON.
WITH BEST WISHES.

James Clark

FEB '08

Getting Your Own Back

"Simply the best book ever written about back pain".
...This compelling book is written in a language that we can all understand"

The Odyssey

James Steele

Published by
Troon Books for Health,
P.O. Box 8566, Troon, Ayrshire, Scotland KA10 7YF

GETTING YOUR OWN BACK
Copyright 2006 © James A Steele

First Published 2006
ISBN: 978-0-9553939-0-7

Published by: Troon Books for Health,
P.O. Box 8566, Troon, Ayrshire, Scotland KA10 7YF

DISCLAIMER
The author and publisher of this material are NOT RESPONSIBLE in any manner whatsoever for any injury which may occur through reading or following the instructions in this manual. The activities, physical or otherwise, described in this material may be too strenuous for some people, and the reader(s) should consult a doctor or physician before engaging in any of them.

Printed by Walker & Connell Ltd., Hastings Square, Darvel
Ayrshire, Scotland, KA17 ODS

CONTENTS

		Page
Foreword		7
Acknowledgements		9
Introduction		11
1	The beginning	13
2	Growing up	17
3	The origin of my bad back and other matters	25
4	Pain	31
5	Marriage	37
6	Sex (with a bad back)	46
7	My phantom ulcer	53
8	A stupid person	59
9	Golf	69
10	Work	88
11	Emergency exercises & calming muscle spasm	102
12	Bad backs - the GP's point of view	111
13	And here's what we do in bed	116
14	Surgery and disc removal	127
15	Muscle spasm	132
16	Its all in the mind	143
17	Lifting, sitting, standing, sleeping	156
18	Exercises	169
19	The importance of 'warm ups' for sport	188
20	Good eating and healthy foods	192
21	The importance of drinking water	205
22	Chinese medicine, acupuncture, chiropractic and others	211
23	Did God have a bad back?	216
24	The Holy Grail Page	227

FOREWORD

James Steele had a mid life crisis soon after his 45th birthday. Arguably, his was more serious than most. After years of chronic back pain, doctors told him his condition could not be treated by further medical intervention. He would just have to learn to live with it, cope by using pain relief and get around by wheelchair if personal mobility was absolutely essential.

James reached rock bottom that day. He had finally run out of solutions. A small army of doctors, osteopaths and chiropractors had kept him going, patching him up for a day, a week, maybe a few months at best. What he did not realise was that treatments like cortisone injections were actually making him worse. Like footballers and sportspeople of a generation ago, he was masking the pain rather than dealing with its underlying cause.

A successful business as a quantity surveyor was about to go down the toilet, as was the great life style he had with it. He had worked hard to achieve it. He might have felt different if his bad back had been the result of an exciting life as a stuntman or through an accident. But his life had been quite ordinary and uneventful in a quiet town on the Ayrshire coast in Scotland. He played golf regularly, looked after the garden and enjoyed the normal rough and tumble with his kids. Rugby had been a great passion as a young man although without any big mishaps or injuries. Yet here he was with a crippling disability.

He tried to live life as normally as possible, in between periods when he could not get out of his house or drive his car. A rare visit to his local golf club, and his life changed suddenly and very much for the better. The club professional mentioned, as an aside almost, that there was someone visiting the area who sorted backs. It was a spur of the moment thing. James had never been a believer in alternative therapies.

In fact he had to be persuaded by his doctors that a course of acupuncture, a visit to the osteopath or chiropractor might be a good idea, especially when he had no idea where else to turn. He was sceptical but desperate at the same time. Was this to be his 'Holy Grail'?

After five sessions with this visiting therapist he could put his socks on. Not the world's greatest achievement, but to him it was like climbing Mount Everest. He recalls that it was truly a life-changing event. He could hardly believe the difference it made. He bombarded his therapist with questions about how the treatment worked, and why it was not more widely known. This book is a story of the events leading to and resulting from that significant moment which irrevocably changed his very existence.

ACKNOWLEDGEMENTS

Sheila,
my wonderful wife!

In times when I was grumpy with back pain, or indeed other times when I was just a stupid thoughtless man, I thank her for turning the other cheek. I thank her for her faith in God and for her faith in me that I could write this book. She has the heart and soul of an angel. Without her I could not have managed many a day when dressing myself or performing the every day chores of ordinary life which were nigh impossible. I have no doubt that some day she will be up there somewhere on a cloud, happy with God by her side. I just hope that I am fortunate to be there with her.

Deborah and Anthony are my darling children. I am greatly indebted for their advice and help on various matters.

Thomas Abrose Bowen, Gene Dobkin and V.S. Ramachandran for the inspiration.

Stuart Bickerstaff, the best friend that I ever had. He gave me the boot up the backside to get the book finished. I miss him so much.

The words of wisdom as applied in various forms by all of the above allowed me to find my Holy Grail.

Additionally my grateful thanks to:

Sandra Malcolm for proof reading and grammar checks.

Kilmarnock Barassie Golf Club for the use of facilities.

I have personally benefited from the therapy administered by James Steele as have some of my patients. This has resulted in great improvement in my symptoms, and an improvement in my general health.

Mr Steele is most professional in his manner and is an excellent communicator. I would have no hesitation in returning to him for treatment. I fully support his endeavours in the exploration of alternative strategies within medicine, where a holistic approach has shown better results than simply treating one aspect of an individual patient's problems.

Dr A Grant McHattie MB ChB MRCGP
Troon, Scotland

I have known James Steele for over 5 years. He has helped me on a number of occasions. He is a man of high integrity and a devotee and expert in Bowen Therapy. I wholeheartedly support him in his endeavours to establish a clinic for research. Although many people do not know exactly how these complimentary therapies work, many of the medical profession now realise they have a place in the management of patients.

J R Anderson FRCS
Consultant Surgeon
South Glasgow
University Hospitals Division
Scotland

INTRODUCTION

The sharp steel of the surgeon's blade glistened. It reflected the sweat on his brow. One slip of the knife, and I would be paralysed for life. Bookmakers don't give odds in this high-risk business. The evening before my inevitable surgery, a worried man, sleep was out of the question. Is there a God out there? Why do I have to suffer as I do? Is it time for retribution? Have I really been such a bad person? No, I was not about to have surgery on my back. Only a fool would allow it. And, yes it was a dream, but sadly my bad back was not.

I have done a lot of ridiculous things in my life, which have hurt my back. This book is a story not just of my mishaps, but a wander with me through life. A story of how my bad back has ruled my existence and how I have come to terms with it. It is the account of my quest for the Holy Grail.

Just where did it all go wrong? Was it an accident in my early life, stupidity in my later life, a sports injury, or was I born with it? How have I treated my body during its life? What effect has my life had on my bad back?

I suffered with chronic back pain for most of my life, and yet did not know the reason why. My life has been a succession of trips to 'quacks' who all offered a cure for back pain. Each time at a new practitioner, I went in the hope that at last there would be something which would rid me of the torture that increased in severity, as I aged. Some of it worked for a while, others were just a complete waste of money. Sadly, it was only after expending copious amounts of the folding variety that I eventually came to the conclusion that I was yet again at the mercy of another Cassandra, who was only in the game for the money.

The public are at the mercy of this type of character. If you are ill, you will search for a cure and will grasp at any kind of treatment, no matter how weird. The chance of finding something to aid your healing is too good to miss. When your life begins each day with a struggle to complete the simple task of putting on your own socks, how can you not yearn for a panacea?

Today, I am middle aged. I have experienced more or less every type of manipulation that exists in my search for a 'cure' for back pain. The word 'cure' of course does not exist. The man who cured people died two thousand years ago. But, we can all get help!

With this experience, I hope that I am able in this book to pass on the advice that I have gleaned. I hope that you will agree that I have completed the task in a light-hearted manner and have written the words in layman's terms that you can all understand. This book will tell of my chance finding that gave me a solution to my back problems. I hope that it will do the same for you.

Chapter One

THE BEGINNING

Books which have been written about 'bad backs' have in common the certainty that they are full of medical jargon. They are often complex, intricate, and downright difficult to read. One's mind struggles to understand the complex jargon used. It would have to be my opinion that they are never written with the reader in mind. Despite this I have over the years bought many of them.

I have often wondered about the authors. Did any of them actually have a bad back? Did they understand how it is, when the top half of your body is in full working order, as is the bottom half, but the hinge in the middle is broken? It is more than a little frustrating when you cannot get both bits to work in conjunction with each other. Suffering as I was with this affliction, I have to admit that I have often vented my irritation with swear words that would make a vicar blush. The books I have read on the subject, coupled with the problems with my own back were the catalyst for this tale.

Thus, I will try to tell the story of my life with chronic back pain.

I have lived with it with difficulty and little by little I have come to terms with it. I have searched the world for something that would restore my health. Often I was frustrated to find a treatment purporting to be my cure-all that was yet one more false dawn. At times I felt suicidal. Ending my life seemed the only answer. Then, as you will read, I found a therapy that worked. It solved all of my problems. Now I live a real, active and pain free life. By reading this book I hope that you may gain some knowledge and understanding of your own back pain. Follow my example and you too can have the same pain free life.

I was born in 1948 in Ardrossan, a small town, in the west coast of Scotland. In time I was joined by one sister and then another. The family, as we thought, was complete. It remained thus for nearly eight years. Then we all got a surprise. I returned from school one day to be greeted by my father, who introduced me to my new brother. I was flabbergasted. Never did I think that we were about to have an addition to the family. At the time I remember thinking that my mother was ill. Her pregnancy was not a topic for discussion at the tea table. I have the feeling that she wanted to keep it a secret. The birds and bees were something we learned from the other kids on the street. Sex education in the home or at school did not exist. However the arrival of my new brother gave much joy. Thus we had four in the family.

I had to come to terms with him. I was eleven when he arrived. I remember saying "He's not going to be sharing my bed." Of course in due time he did. The age gap meant that I never really got to grips with teaching him all of the things that a good brother should have, but eventually I came to love him. Today he is one of my best friends. I would do anything for him.

My father was missing from our house for long periods. He spent his time at sea as an engineering officer. He was often far from home; indeed at times he would be on the other side of the world. My father earned good wages. As a family we were pretty well off. There was enough to eat and a comfortable home. We were fortunate to own one of the few cars that existed in our town. Looking back I can see that we had no financial difficulties although it was not something that I gave consideration to at the time. My mother knew how to manage her husband and her children, giving them a secure and happy home. However, I could recognise that at times she was exhausted trying to raise the family on her own. Eventually the time came when she could take it no longer. My father had to stop his wanderings and look for a shore job.

Ardrossan was a busy seaport at the time and had a thriving shipyard. Thankfully it was in need of an experienced engineer. Thus my father took up employment there and, skilled in engineering and man management, he was quickly promoted to a senior position. The shipyard at that time employed about six hundred workers. We lived in Glasgow Street, the longest street in Ardrossan. A boulevard or avenue it wasn't, a great length of straight faceless tarmac it was. I was often awakened at seven thirty in the morning by the clunk of the steel shod boots that all of the men wore as they walked past our house on the way to 'The Yard'.

The yard built fine ships, many of them for the cargo and passenger lines which plied across the sea from Scotland to Ireland. Ardrossan in those days had a number of shipping lines that used the port: Burns & Laird and Coast Lines and others. Most sailed to Belfast, Larne and Londonderry on a daily basis, going out with supplies and returning with fine produce from the Irish fields.

The harbour was a dirty and dusty place, busy in the export of coal to Ireland, which having no coal had to import it. Most of their supplies came from the Ayrshire coalmines. The coal came to the docks by rail. It was loaded on wagons straight from the pits and then transported to the waiting ships in the harbour. Special cranes at the dockside lifted the wagons. They were turned on their side and the contents dropped straight into the gaping holds of the cargo boats. Kelly was the name of the Belfast shipping line which did most of this work. Twenty years later when I next visited Belfast, I was pleased to see the coal merchant still existed.

As a lad I spent a lot of my spare time at the harbour. There was much to see. Metal plate from the Motherwell steel and rolling mills was regularly exported from the port. It was heading for the famous

Belfast shipyard of Harland and Wolf, where they were the builders of many great liners, 'Titanic' perhaps the most readily remembered.

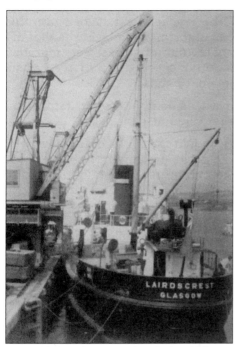

A ship in Ardrossan Harbour in the 1950's loading and unloading cargo.

Standing at the dockside I did often wonder what would happen if a big wave came over a ship carrying a load of steel plate and swamped it. With a cargo of such density would it go to the bottom of the sea?

Sadly, some years later a small ship, the 'Lairdsfield' was lost on her way to Belfast, loaded with flat steel plate. The crew of ten perished. I am no expert, but I suppose that one minute she would be pushing through the waves and perhaps a hatch cover came loose. The waves crashing over would have filled the hold in seconds. The crew would have had no chance of reaching life jackets or even sending out a mayday signal.

The estuary of the river Clyde is littered with wrecks. It is a dangerous life at sea. I suppose that few of us accept the fact that even with the increasing use of airfreight, most of the food we eat still comes to us by sea. An awful lot of men and today women too, are risking their lives at sea as we sleep.

Shipyards in those days had little in the way of mechanical aids. Much of the lifting and moving was done with the sweat and donkeywork of the labourers who had all of the menial tasks to complete. I wonder how many of them today have bad backs. Perhaps though their daily toils gave them fitness and a muscle strength that few of us have today? Maybe they never suffered with back pain?

I don't think that I was a troublesome boy; however my mother may have another opinion. Our home was very much a puritan ménage where regular attendance at church was expected. I have to say that I was not much in favour of it and objected to being forced to go. I attended a fairly solid school, which fulfilled its aim of providing the basics in education. I don't think that it sent out any imperial administrators, businessmen, writers or theologians although I seem to remember that a few of its inmates made it eventually to Glasgow University and beyond.

At school I was unspeakably bored. The school taught Latin, French and Mathematics to those intending to progress to a higher level of education. I was more interested in art, woodwork and technical subjects. I enjoyed working with my hands and was creative. I was frequently late for school and consequently suffered punishment in the form of that famous Scottish hand warmer - the tawse! – a long piece of hardened leather, which the teacher kept, folded over his shoulder under his tunic. Those of us unfortunate to be late (and it did seem that the same faces were pretty regular attendees) were marched to the teachers' office, where we would be lined up to receive six whacks of the brute on the palms of cold hands.

I often protested my innocence with a long and often fantastical explanation for my lateness, but was belted just the same.

Growing up I became old enough to join the ranks of the boys who had unofficial summer jobs down the docks. Ireland in those days was a great place for holidays. Many Scottish people were only too glad to take a trip across the water. The harbour in Ardrossan had two stations, where steam trains would arrive at regular intervals just before the ships were due to sail. The trains would be loaded with passengers from Glasgow, who were already in holiday mood and in fine fettle having probably consumed their fair share of alcohol on the train journey. The passengers would thus alight on the platform to be met by our group of wee boys who would shout out "carry your case, mister?"

Those about to go on holiday did feel a bit posh and as a result the last thing that they wanted to do was to carry their own suitcase from the train to the gangplank at the ship. Thus I was often to be seen breathlessly trying to carry suitcases that sometimes were as big as me. Off I would go puffing and panting with a bit of really heavy luggage at the end of each straining arm. The reward for this toil, if you were lucky, could be as much as two and sixpence. (12.5p in today's terms). A quick "thank you sir," and I would sprint back to the train to see if I could find another customer.

I was a small thin youth then. Thinking about it now I have often wondered what this strenuous lifting did to my back. But at the time my only goal was to earn money and the damage that I may have been doing to my back was of little consequence. What little pain I had at the time I ignored.

Things were different in those days: much safer. I don't ever remember my mother worrying about me getting home after midnight, walking all the way on my own in the poorly lit streets. There were always a few drunks rolling home from some illicit drinking den at that time of night.   .

The pubs in Scotland in those days all closed at ten o'clock, but even the local bobby (police officer) could find somewhere to have a fly pint of beer after hours. The back door of many an establishment was left ajar just for this purpose. Ardrossan though was a safe place to live and it was well policed.

Chapter Two

GROWING UP

When I was aged fourteen my mother was ill with Pleurisy. Indeed at one point she came close to death. But thanks to the skill of the physicians and the help of the Lord, she got better. I am happy to say that she is still with us today. When she was ill in hospital, our family had no matriarch to guide us and thus the family was split up. My two sisters went to live with an aunt and uncle in a modern house at the top end of the town. It was a comfortable residence complete with central heating and other comforts. My father and I went to live with his rather aged parents, in their old house located next to the harbour.

This house had high ceilings, and draughty windows. The heating system consisted of a black grate in the front parlour where my grandfather would light a fire in the mornings. It was not much of a life for my dad and me. If was worse for my grandfather who had to go out in all weathers to split sticks for kindling and then carry in buckets of coal. I would often stare out of the window in the front of the house at the cargo ships that would be docked in the harbour and wonder which part of the world they had come from.

Sometimes I would wander down the docks and sit on the bollards that held the ropes securing the ships to the jetty. The system for unloading cargo in those days did not have the safe handling procedures that we take for granted today. Hessian bags and wooden boxes of all sorts of sizes sat precariously on a wood and rope arrangement that could hardly be described as high-tech. Then one of the big grey cranes that were situated every 100 yards around the dock-side would swing the pallets of cargo over my head as it was being unloaded from the ships. Sitting as I did I gave little consideration to my safety.

In those days the harbour employed a good number of men in the capacity as 'dock labourer'. These fellows had to climb down into the hold of the ships and manually load the bags and boxes onto the pallets. I gave no thought to the fact that at least some of them must have suffered with back pain. Of course there were no manual handling instructions, safety helmets or indeed any form of personal safety equipment that is the norm today. The men were of all sizes. The fellow who lived next to my grandparents had such a job. He was of Irish descent as were most of the fellows who did these manual tasks. He wasn't a big fellow, so I have no idea how he managed to heave all of these heavy packets. I do though remember that he had seven children. So the job although exhausting must have left him with some energy for later in the day!

Between visits to the hospital to see my mother, my father continued with his duties at the shipyard so most of the time I was left to my own devices. I was bored and I didn't like living in the house with people who were so old. My grandfather was a lovely man but my grandmother was difficult to live with. I preferred to stay out of the house as long as possible. It was vexatious to say the least when I went to my second home at the end of each school day. The summer holidays were looming and I knew that it would be difficult to cope. I discussed the matter with my father and he said that he would do what he could to find me a summer job.

Burns & Laird, the Glasgow shipping line, engaged the shipyard at Ardrossan for the repair of their vessels. My father had become friendly with their superintendent. He had a word with the man to see if he could pull a few strings and find me a summer job on one of their ships. A boy going to sea in those days had to be sixteen years of age. Although I was just fourteen, I suppose that I must have looked older. My father is not the kind of man who would tell a lie. So I suppose that he must have conveniently sidestepped the question of age had it come into the equation.

Thus he secured my first wage-paying occupation - washing dishes in the pantry of the First Class restaurant on the M.V. 'Irish Coast.' My official title was - Pantry Boy.

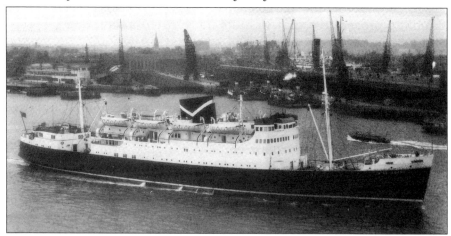

M.V. 'Irish Coast' The ship sailed from Ardrossan to Belfast from May to September each year.

The vessel was a passenger ship, which made a return trip to Belfast every day during the summer months. Built at the Harland and Wolf shipyard in Belfast, of 3,324 tons displacement, A1 at Lloyds, she represented a step forward in technical development in that she was one of the first vessels to be converted to carry motorcars: a precursor to the drive on/drive off vessels we take for granted today. In the winter months she would carry passengers in the comfortable cabins of the upper decks. Below she would carry cattle. In the summer the cattle decks were cleaned out and the space made ready for passenger traffic. A lift which lowered the cars for storage below decks was fitted on the deck ahead of the bridge. The lift could accommodate four cars at a time and thus it would take some while to stow the fifty or so cars which travelled with us each day.

Northern Ireland in those days was a popular place for holidays

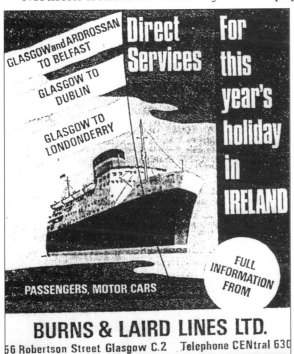

and accordingly, the little ship often carried a full complement. She was designed for relief work on the shipping routes from Scotland and England to Ireland and was used in the winter to take the place of other ships when they went for annual refit. Consequently she had no regular route of her own, except that is for the summer season, sailing out of Ardrossan.

The ship was rather unsuitable for her summer occupation. Good quality cabins in First Class located to the front of the ship took up about two thirds of the vessel, but most folk in those days could not afford the luxury of a first class ticket. Those who did had room to wander at their leisure. In the Second Class at the back of the ship, some days we would have over fifteen hundred holidaymakers. They were happy, but squashed into the least amount of space, with most of them below decks, spending their time imbibing at the temporary construction that served as a bar.

The bar was a converted steel container with some fold-down serving hatches. It sat on a canvas hatch cover under which and out of sight were yet more cattle pens. Around it the steel decks were cleaned and painted red. A number of sofas were placed around the deck to give the appearance that it was always such. The passengers on the first day of their annual holiday were more interested in guzzling booze that taking any notice of the tell-tales signs which indicated that this area of the ship was recently converted from stock-pens for the cattle that the ship carried in winter months.

However, there I was happily at sea on a lovely ship. Looking back, the ship seemed huge as she sat at the quay-side in Ardrossan. In reality when compared with some of the massive ships we have today she was tiny. On the crossing from Ardrossan to Belfast we sailed down the wide estuary of the River Clyde. Then we would venture out into the open bit of sea between Scotland and Ireland known as the North Channel.

Some days the sea would be rough. Many passengers would be sea-sick. I must have had my dad's sea-legs as the bad weather never bothered me.

As the pantry boy in the First Class (kitchen), my task was to wash the mountains of dishes that were used in the First Class restaurant. Bent as I was, over a sink for long hours, is perhaps another contributing factor to the back problems I have today. Yet as I worked on the ship, the pain in my back was something that I gave little regard to.

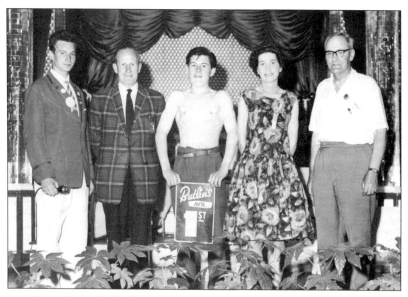

James winning the Mr Muscles competition at Butlin's Holiday camp. Circa 1960

It came and went. It was as far as I was concerned just part of the job. Did we not all have sore backs at some time or other? The Able Seamen who worked the decks hauling the ropes and other such manual tasks did not seem to mind the physicality of their chores, nor did they complain of backache.

Perhaps hard manual work gave strength to the larger back muscles that protected the weaker ones?

On the ship, I was a slip of a lad. Ten stone seven pounds in my socks, and not a bit of fat on me. Fit as a flea. Running about the decks, loading stores in the morning, washing multitudes of dishes, cleaning bits of the ship and all of my other allotted chores kept me fit. I never gave a thought to my old age and what kind of condition my back would be in later life.

The bonus that I had working on the ship was that I had accommodation aboard in a cabin that I shared with three other lads. This allowed me some freedom and saved me from having to live with my grandparent's in their draughty old house. Allowing though that the work that we had to do was considered the lowest-of-the-low our cabin was to the same standard. Thus we were stuck in a room located on the lowest deck and next to the engine room. It had no portholes and we had to rely on air that came through pipes in a sort of old-fashioned conditioning system. It was hot.

However as far as I was concerned it was heaven! The summer season lasted six weeks and I considered it six weeks of bliss.

The working day commenced at 6.30am, when we would be awoken by the Second Steward, a fellow called Archie McLaughlin. He had a touch of humour, or so he thought. I could hear him taking great delight, banging on doors to awaken the crew, who slept in cabins situated along an alleyway adjacent to us. Some of the men who worked on the ship were fond of a beer or two. The ship, on her return from Belfast would dock in Ardrossan at 8.00pm.

After unloading the cars, and letting the passengers ashore, it didn't leave a lot of time to get to the pub that was located nearest to the harbour. Allowing that pubs in those days had a licence to serve alcohol until just 10.00pm, it was always a bit of a sprint up the dock road to get there as quickly as possible. This would allow the crew members an hour and a half or so to quench their thirst, during which much beverage would be consumed. Of course many of the pubs and bars didn't abide by the rules, and would allow some illegal after-hours drinking. Thus at times, very late in the evening, I could often hear the older crew members returning to the ship, and imbibed as they were, very much worse for wear.

Amazingly at muster first thing in the morning they would be bright as a button.

In my second season on the ship, I was given promotion to the position of pantry boy, in one of the two Second Class restaurants, which I gladly accepted. It may seem strange that I considered a move from the First to the Second Class a promotion, but the simple fact was that there I had to look after all that happened with food production in the restaurant. In a way, I was my own boss, which was pleasing. The responsibility allowed that I had not just the task of washing the dishes, but had to help setting the tables, and additionally had to dash back and forth across the deck from the restaurant to the main galley in the ship, to fetch the hot food that was sold in the restaurant. The galley was located next to the First Class pantry where I had worked in my first year on the vessel.

The menu in the restaurant was banal to say the least. Not that the passengers knew, but the same choice of food repeated in the restaurant every day, throughout the summer season. It consisted of soup of the day followed by a choice of cold salmon or roast beef, or a hot dish of grilled fish. All served with potatoes and peas. Then there was a choice of apple pie, or jelly and meringue, washed down with copious amounts of strong dark tea. Carrying the pots and pans full of food, from the galley, out over the open decks to my restaurant at the rear of the ship, kept me fit. The strong muscles that I still have in my fore-arms are a result of carrying the heavy pans day after day. These sturdy muscles have held me in good stead through the years. They were able to help me with the building work on the homes that we have had. Even today they are helping me, when I have time for a game of golf, where holding the club tightly when controlling the flight of the ball is so important. However, to return to the story:

The following year I was promoted once again, with this time the reward of the position of Second Steward in the Second Class bar. There I worked with a nice man, a fellow called Willie Anderson. He hailed from Saltcoats, a town next to Ardrossan. He taught me all that there was to know about serving alcoholic beverages. One down-side to the position was the fact that we had to go ashore to collect the barrels of beer and Guinness, left for us on the quay-side. This was heavy work that hurt my back. However, Willie taught me a lifting procedure that helped reduce the risk. He explained how to put one hand on the barrel and the other on his shoulder. He then put his hand on the other side of the barrel with his other hand on my shoulder. Thus we had a sort of suspension system where we were able to lift the barrel and suspend it between us.

The barrels were heavy and we had to stagger in this format down the gangplank onto the ship, and then down a flight of stairs, to the bar located in the deck below. Cantilevering the barrels between us allowed that we could lift them, but the huge weight we carried between us undoubtedly had a contribution to my back problems in later years. I doubt that an employer today would allow its operatives to carry things in such a manner. Yet in those days, we had no mechanised fork-lifts and such to help when lifting.

I have lots of stories that I could tell about my times on the boat. I learned much about life. In all it was a jolly time. There is much to tell, but perhaps these humorous tales are best left for my next book. Nonetheless, one thing that did change my life that I will mention, was meeting Sheila, the woman who was later to become my wife, and later in life my crutch, at times of need, when my back pain was excruciating.

My early years on board ship were a learning curve. Girls were something that existed, but I was more interested in making some money to see me through the winter, when pocket-money may be scarce. By the fourth year on the ship, I was older and wiser and began to take an interest in the girls who came to work with us.

The Irish Coast employed six girls, who worked in the First Class restaurant. In the mornings and again in the afternoon, they would serve the passengers who would come to the restaurant for tea and cakes. In between, the girls would take turns to serve in the Tea Bar, located in an alleyway to the side of the Pursers office. All of the crew on the ship looked forward to seeing these girls come aboard.

Invariably they would be good-looking specimens, fresh from completing school works at Ardrossan Academy. The boys, who worked at various tasks on the ship, would try to befriend one or other of them.

But I was then a pale skinny fellow with a spotty face. Never did I assume that I would have a chance of cultivating a relationship with any of them. Despite this, I would often find an excuse to wander up to the tea bar for chat. Resplendent as I was in black trousers, white tunic with a row of polished brass buttons up the front, and blue shoulder epaulettes with the ships badge etched in silver thread, I at least looked the part. Although I would laugh and joke with all of the girls, I had admiration for just one.

Little by little, I found that Sheila would find some of her spare time to come and visit me, in the Second Class bar where I worked. Our friendship grew. Then one day I took the courage to ask if she would come out with me for the evening. By then, I was eighteen. I had passed my driving test, and my dad was willing (reluctantly) to allow me to have the use of his car. Thus one evening, after the ship docked in the harbour, I was a happy and proud man with my new girl-friend beside me, as we drove though the Ayrshire countryside, and north to the coastal town of Largs, which in those days was a nice place to visit.

There, I took Sheila to the best hotel in the town, where I bought her a gin and tonic or whatever was her tipple in those days. We laughed and shared good conversation. Later we had a walk along the beach. I can remember that my heart was thumping as I pondered on whether or not she would allow me to hold her hand. Of course she did. I was pleased to be walking along holding the hand of such a lovely girl and pleased to have such a nice person for a friend.

The closeness with Sheila developed. At times, as I suppose as with any young couple, the relationship was turbulent. Despite this we grew to love each other. Eventually my mum told me that either I should think of getting married to the girl or getting on with the rest of my life. Thankfully I made the decision to ask for her hand in marriage.

But for the chance of my mother being ill, my father finding me a job on the ship and Sheila taking the place of her sister (who had decided to pull out of the job at the last minute) we might never have met. God indeed was good to organise such a complexity of events that have allowed this chance meeting to develop into a bond that has now lasted so many happy years.

My times on the Irish Coast were an important part of my growing up. The work on the ship was a revelation at times! An education certainly! A contributing factor to my back pain in later life – who knows!

Chapter Three

THE ORIGIN OF MY BAD BACK and OTHER MATTERS

I cannot really remember when it all started. The odd jobs that I did as a lad did not help. These various part-time activities required me at times to bend my back and to lift heavy objects. There is no doubt I gave little care to the proper way that one should lift things. No one thought to give me instruction how to do so. And, of course, I didn't have the brains to ask. Very few of us did in those days. We just got on with it no matter the consequences. Of course, once you have a bad back you become careful to assume the correct position when picking up heavy objects. Now like a reformed smoker I probably do more than my fair share of lecturing to others on the correct procedures.

Apart from the work on the ship in the summer months, I remember having a job at a railway station. In the sidings lay the coal wagons to be unloaded. There were no mechanical shovels in those days. Everything was done manually. Employment for a big strapping, fit man! One with muscles! Not a job for the puny weakling who presented himself for service one Easter holiday period. It must have looked that there was more to my framework when I was clothed. I am sure that if the foreman had seen me stripped he would never have considered offering me the position.

The job was the dirtiest and hardest I have ever undertaken. The shovel, which I was supposed to use to lift the coal lumps, was as big as me. I was expected to empty the coal wagons and load the dirty black lumps into coal bags. It was a difficult task. Each had to weigh one hundredweight (50kg) when filled. The balancing act clipping the edge of the sack to the weigh machine and then filling with coal was an art. Often the bag would fall from the machine when it was only half full. The damage to my vertebrae as I struggled to re-attach it to the mechanism was anyone's guess.

I was expected to fill fifty sacks per day but the work was so exhausting that my energy level ran out long before the day came an end. I don't think that I ever reached the daily target. The foreman allowed me two days to get the hang of things but after three days I think he could see that I was struggling to cope. On the fourth day he had a quiet word in my ear and suggested that the next day would be my last. So the job lasted just a week, but it gained me quite a bit of cash that was valuable to a poor student.

I should have spent a bit of the money on washing soap. I certainly had to use copious amounts each evening. In those days not many of us had a shower in the home. Thus I had to fill a bath to have a scrub. Half way through I would have to get out of it dripping wet. I would then empty the water from the bath, clean the bath of all of the coal dust which was now stuck to the sides, refill it, get back in and continue washing. Soaking in the tub while I did this gave some solace to my back pain. I suppose I thought that this back pain was just a consequence of the job. Never did I consider that I might have some structural weakness.

I know now, but didn't understand in my early days that the human body is a remarkable piece of equipment. It consists mostly of water. Indeed we are 70 % water. (The brain is 80% water – blood 92%) Thus our skeletal frame floats in the water of our bodies. It has the task not just of holding us upright but also of protecting our vital organs. The skull protects the brain. The rib cage protects the respiratory system. The pelvis protects the reproductive organs. But in essence our skeletal frame is simply a coat hanger for the muscles.

The bones in our bodies are composed of half water and half solid matter. They contain nearly two pounds of calcium and more than a pound of phosphorus. That is enough phosphorus for two thousand match heads. If we look at the skeleton (pictured here) we will see that above the pelvic girdle and below the ribcage we find part of the vertebral column, which consists of just five vertebrae. These lumbar vertebrae are a set of bones separated by pads. The pads are discs of cartilage that act as shock absorbers when we move. This and the bones in a line above it are called the spine or spinal column. Allowing that bones will go where muscles put them, my skeletal frame was often contorted when the muscles went into painful spasm and pulled me out of shape.

There are six hundred and thirty nine named muscles in the human body. Yet in the time of Galen (130-

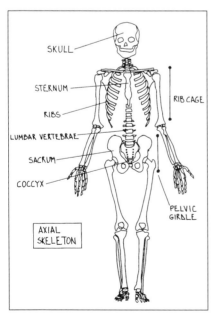

A human skeleton

200), one of the first great anatomists, few of the muscles had names. It was not largely until the 18th century, thanks to English anatomist William Cowper and Scottish anatomist James Douglas, that the specific myological terminology we use today was established. Fortunately quite a few of these muscles are arranged around the vertebral column, which as you can see has not a lot to support it, but takes an awful lot of strain during our daily lives.

I think that it is remarkable that the human body was designed in such a way. God, or who-ever it was who did the designing, made a great job. But not all of us are born with all of our bits in the correct place. Sometimes, indeed we can have an extra rib. Others of us are born with deficiencies.

I have a hairy naevus over the lower part of my back - a little bunch of fine hairs that grow at the base of the spine and can cover an area the size of a saucer. This can be a sign of a mild form of spina bifida. Apparently a lot of us have it. It is not something to worry about so don't go looking at yourself in the mirror, especially if you have not had any real back pain. I always knew that I had this hairy bit on my back. As a lad I probably never gave it much thought, although I do remember some of my friends at the swimming pool remarking about it. As it was so prominent I have wondered why not one doctor ever explained to me what it was.

Spina bifida in its worst form is known to be a developmental defect in which the newborn baby is born with part of its spinal chord and its covering exposed through a gap in the backbone. Thankfully I have a very mild form of this. It is known as spina bifida occulta. With this there is a defect in the bony arch of the spine that (unlike spina bifida) has a normal skin covering and, as I have, there may be an overlaying hairy patch. Recent evidence suggests that the risk of spina bifida is reduced if extra folic acid (a vitamin of the B group, present in all green plants) is included in the diet of pregnant women in the first three months of pregnancy. As I was born not many years after the Second World War I suppose that there may have been a lack of such vegetables. I had good parents who gave me the best food that was available at the time. We ate no rubbish. The research into spina bifida simply hadn't happened until many years later. The findings of an incidental x-ray explained at least in part the reason for my continual back pain.

Making money was always an important part of my life. The spare time jobs were a must. In-between I would play some rugby (more stress on the spine) and add in a bit of time on the golf course. Later in life I worked hard creating a business. This involved a lot of hours behind a desk, or behind the wheel of the car, driving to numerous meetings. None of this was in any way good for my back.

When my toils with the business were in full flow I was by then disinclined to exercise. Work was all encompassing. My body needed some time to unwind and relax from the tensions of its daily toils. As a result, I exacerbated my back problem. I was not willing to accept the simple principle that exercise strengthens and tones the muscles. Consequently, I would have times of excruciating back pain. Happening at regular intervals, this caused me to miss many days at work. (Indeed, it is said that more workdays are lost to back problems than the common cold). For that reason my back pain progressed from a simple ailment to a chronic back problem and was beginning to change my life.

Due partly to physical discomfort and restricted back movement, it was more than just periods of pain and stiffness. Visits to the doctor and the temporary relief from the painkillers he dispensed only masked the injuries. Bed rest or periods flat on my back on the floor, I am sure only further weakened my back. Poor body posture resulted. Lying around on a sofa like a Roman centurion, with a host of nubile women attending to your every whim, will in time cause the back to grow weaker. Of course, I wasn't a centurion and I didn't have any slaves to pamper me, but I did indulge in this kind of slovenly behaviour, collapsing on the sofa at the end of yet another hard day at the office. Thus my back weakened and became yet more vulnerable.

Two of the most common types of musculoskeletal pain are muscle strains and joint injuries. Muscle strains can be caused by overstretching and are usually minor irritations. They can be treated relatively simply. Joint injuries on the other hand, especially in the spine, can be a different problem altogether. Probably I had a combination of both, although the one which obviously caused me more pain was the damage done to my vertebral column.

Often the nerves exciting the injured joint became inflamed, irritated, or pinched. This in turn seemed to give me pain in other parts of my body. At times it would radiate down either or both legs. I now know that this is called referred pain. In other words it radiates down the body from the affected area. In the lower limbs it is often referred to as sciatica. I often had this kind of discomfort. It is a persistent pain in the area of the sciatic nerve and is usually felt down the back and outer side of the thigh, calf and foot. It can be continuous all the way down, or it can manifest itself just at points down the leg.

The sciatic nerve is the principal nerve of the lower limb and is formed in the pelvis from branches of several of the lumbar and sacral spinal nerves. It passes below the sacroiliac joint (the joint on either side of the five fused vertebrae at the base of the spine that form the sacrum – just above the coccyx) to the buttock, then behind the hip joint to the back of the thigh. It is deeply buried in muscles throughout its course. Above the knee it divides into branches, which between them supply all the structures below the knee. Sciatica is a symptom and not a disease and in each case it is the cause of the problem that has to be identified and treated and not the sciatica itself. The onset may be sudden, brought on by an awkward lifting or twisting movement, which can cause pressure on a spinal nerve, usually by an invertebral (slipped disc). Sometimes it can be caused by pressure on the nerve in the thigh from a bad sitting posture or a badly designed seat.

Working in my office for long hours tied to a desk I often had this type of soreness. Back then, of course, I did not know what was wrong, just that I was hurting. When I knew nothing, or indeed very little about my sore back, all I could do to help this type of pain was to rest and take mouthfuls of painkillers. It was initially the only thing that would help, but as you will see, eventually I found other ways to assist.

The question that most back pain sufferers ask is - how does it happen? I suppose that there must be many reasons but in my youth I simply didn't know the answer. The days I spent as a lad in my various works certainly did me no favours. My Easter holiday unloading the coal wagons exhausted not just my back but my whole body. Almost certainly the source of my back pain was when I was particularly stupid in attempting to lift heavy objects. Then the pain receptors in my body would click into gear.

Pain receptors send a signal to the spinal column, up to the brain and back again at some three hundred metres per second. This is known as the feed-back loop system. The brain itself doesn't have any pain receptors but does the receipting of pain from other parts of the body, analyses it and makes it obvious that you are hurt.

Pain receptors in the body will gradually adapt to the poor structural spinal alignment that it has to cope with. If, for example you push your finger back far enough to feel a pull, this will mirror how a joint feels when it is overstretched. If you were to leave the finger in that position for weeks you would eventually feel less pain. (I don't recommend it though.) The nerve receptors would have been over stimulated and thus would be sending fewer messages to the brain. Thus the body adapts. As a lad though, I knew little of this!

And so the beginnings of my back pain just sort of crept up on me. Little by little the back muscle spasms and the pain that went with it started to take over my life.

Chapter Four

PAIN

Pain is like a voice over a telephone wire as it zooms from an injured area along a network of nerves. Each nerve carries different messages. Nerves join together to make nerve bundles. Some carry pain. Others carry temperature and position messages. I suppose that's why when we have pain, we can also have numbness, tingling and hot and cold spots. Nobody likes pain, but pain is vital to the human protective mechanism. Without this ability to experience pain, we would cause our bodies more damage. It is the body's defensive apparatus and its method of telling you that something is out of line and needs correcting.

While I was engaged in all of my revenue earning activities in my youth, my body was trying to tell me that all was not well, but I was not equipped to understand what my body was telling me. My body is designed to stay healthy, despite the many abuses I throw at it. Yet when it couldn't cope, it used the pain to let me know that all was not healthy and that something needed attention.

Pain is something that we all fear: a manifestation that we want to avoid at all cost. There may be some silly folk out there who enjoy it, but as far as I am concerned, suffering, distress, ache, discomfort, agony, worry, anguish, and grief are all things that most of us would like to avoid. I pride myself as someone who has half a brain. I know that pain hurts. Thus, I now don't allow myself to get into dangerous situations that would be likely to hurt me.

We all experience pain at some time in our lives. The Bible tells us that Jesus had a very meek and mild manner. There is though no mention of his back pain, if he had such a thing. In crucifixion his pain and suffering by far encompassed anything that the humans on this planet could ever understand.

The writer, a poor mortal, accepts the fact that in life pain is something that we just have to embrace and get on with. In all of the vast numbers now residing on this planet, there could indeed be very few who have not suffered pain of one kind or the other.

Why then when I stupidly injured myself, did I still continue do the same silly things that hurt me? The answer sometimes did make me look a bit brainless. I should have looked after myself better, changed my way of life. But when I was pain-free I became careless and did all sorts of things that I shouldn't. Sometimes I hurt myself simply by bending forward too quickly, perhaps to lift something from the floor, or to unplug the vacuum from a socket at skirting level!

Skirting level sockets are not in a good place for people with bad backs. You would think I would have had the sense to refit all of the electrical sockets and such like in my home, to a level which would not require me to bend. I really did need to change my lifestyle and in turn reduce my risk. I never did though.

There were times when I lived a relatively pain free life. Careful not to hurt myself, I would remember the excruciating pain that I suffered when my back muscles went into awful spasm. But then, as these pain free days drifted by, I gradually forgot and fell into the same old bad habits. A fully fit person can get away with bad habits, but not any of us suffering from back pain. Prior to finding my Holy Grail I had to concentrate and give simple daily chores all of my attention. Thoughtlessly doing something stupid, such as bending forward to hastily retrieve something which had fallen from my grasp was a recipe for disaster. With my back in its pain mode, sleep came fitfully. As a result, I tended to catnap as if on guard. I found this exhausting. Many a morning I would arise more tired that I went to bed the night before. During the night I would drift off from time to time, but I would be afraid to fully let go as more often than not I knew that I would be awakened with a bolt of pain.

One morning, after a somewhat uncomfortable night, tossing and turning, trying to attain a decent sleeping position, I was in waking mode. Listening to classical music on my favourite radio station, it was about seven in the morning, and I was considering emergence from the bedcovers. Without thinking, I turned sharply onto my side, only to knock my back muscles into spasm. My body went into a cold sweat. I knew that it would take some minutes for the pain to die down and that I would also have to spend the remainder of the day in a protective state looking after the muscles that had been hurt. I was very aware of the fact that throughout the day ahead of me one false move, one stupid act and the evil pain would return. I lived in fear but in one way or another survived that day.

The morning after I awoke feeling much better! The trauma of the previous day faded. Cautiously, I used all the correct procedures to get on my feet. I decided to have a shower. The chrome shelving that I had sensibly fitted in the corners of the showers at waist and shoulder level prevented the need to bend for soap or shower gel. I managed to wash without difficulty.

Turning off the water in the shower, I turned and reached for a towel. This simple twisting motion allowed me to slip on the still wet floor. Just an inch or two, yet instantly my back muscles went into spasm. All of them at the one time it seemed. I screamed with pain. Immobilised with my brain whirling I was confused as to what to do. Grabbing the rail above the shower door, I stood trembling and crying until the pain died down. My wife who had heard all of this commotion was now at my side. She tenderly dried me, and gingerly with her help, I put on some clothes.

After my brain cleared, I was able to make some sort of sense of the situation. I thought of the exercises that I had learned for such a crisis. I considered if I would be able to lie on my bed to do them. If I lay down on the bed, would I be able to get back up?

Having done this so many times before, I should be able to cope. Or would I? I was in a quandary. The sensible route would be to attempt the exercises. However, I decided that the risk was too great. The sting of yet more muscle spasm, should I make the wrong move, was just too much of a danger. I took the coward's way out.

The office in my house is just down the corridor from my bedroom. I walked slowly towards it, entered the room and perched on the edge of my office chair. I sat for a minute. Then for no conceivable reason a pain surged down the outside of my right leg. Then I had no idea what it was. Now I know that it was sciatica. Perched on the edge of my chair, I had the feeling that eventually the pain would subside. Feeling better I got up turned and lifted some papers from a shelf. I returned to the seat and sat back down again. The phone rang. I answered. Soon I was engaged in conversation. My brain clicked into gear. The fellow on the other end of the phone knew nothing about backs and even less about the construction problem that he was discussing with me. In full-flow I did my job and explained how he could extricate himself from his dilemma. For a few minutes I forgot all about my back pain. Then that same old sharp jab of pain, as if my spinal column was clicking out of place reminded me to sit up straight. The day wore on. I tried to put the pain out of my mind by busying myself with my writings in the office, making yet more telephone calls and such.

I managed to survive that day and then a few days more. Slowly the pain started to subside. I found though that the more often that I hurt my back, the longer it took to heal. Was this just old age, or was it a sign that the more often I hurt myself, the more carefully I had to look at my life style? Should I be taking things in life just a little bit more slowly? Should I change my job? My furrowed brow grew. I just didn't know the answers.

The cumulative effect of these days with back pain prevented me from enjoying a game of golf. A pastime, very dear to my heart! I have been a member of my golf club for quite a number of years and yet some seasons when my back was bad I hardly had a game. Perhaps I became afraid of hurting myself. Conceivably I did, but then who wants to inflict pain on themselves, especially the kind that lingers for so long whenever you injure yourself. Possibly I just became a coward, trapped in my own little world of self-inflicted pain!

Pain is distinct from other sensations and is carried by its own nerve fibres. Preoccupied, a man may hardly notice an injury that he would find painful at another time. Yet another man who is anxious and expecting pain may feel more pain than the injury is worth. For some people sitting in the dentist's chair can be much like this. All pain is in the mind. It has no other existence. Colours, sounds, smells, textures and so, are things that we are aware of as having a real understanding. They are measurable events around us. Pain has no such counterpart in the real world. However when back muscles are in spasm, pain and the fear that goes with it are very real in one's brain.

Pain provokes various reflex actions of which sweating, nausea and faintness are familiar examples. By disturbing the heart and circulation, pain contributes to shock (failure of the circulation), a sometimes-fatal complication of extensive injury or severe acute illness. Anaesthetics, on the other hand, have made surgery safer as well as less unpleasant and mostly pain free. The Chinese with their own form of acupuncture worked out thousands of years ago that the body will release painkillers (endorphins) if you carefully and precisely place some needles into the area of concern.

An individual can experience painful sensations that are not real. For example, a person may continue to experience pain in an amputated limb. This phantom limb pain is caused by inactivity in the sensory neurons. V. S. Ramachandran, an American M.D. and somewhat of an expert in this subject tells a story about the fellow who worked in a steel plant. The poor man caught his (right) arm in a rolling mill. The man lost the arm, yet after he had healed he could still feel the pain of his fingernails digging into the palm of his hand as the mill tore his arm from him. Needless to say Ramachandran found a way to rid the man of the pain.

Accepting that the right side of the brain controls the left side of the body and vice-versa (more or less), Ramachandran constructed a long box about the length of a man's arm, with a partition down the middle. It had an opening on the right side at one end that allowed the patient to look through, with his right eye looking through its own hole but only down the one partitioned side of the box. At the far end of the box there was a mirror. The man placed his remaining left arm into the box and in the partitioned left side.

As the man looked though the aperture and down the right side of the box, the mirror allowed him to see the arm in the left side. Ramachandran asked the man to close his right eye and then his left hand. Then he asked him to open his right eye and once focused, while looking at the image in the mirror, then to slowly open his left hand. In essence what he was attempting to do was to fool the brain. The optic nerves carry visual information from special sensory receptors in the eyes. These nerves contain about 1 million sensory nerve fibres. Visual information from the lateral half of the left eye and medial half of the right eye go to the left side of the brain, the opposite happening with the other eye.

The subject of what the brain does and how the brain works is a complex topic. Suffice to say that Ramachandran had worked out that by encouraging the man to open his left hand but look at the action only with the right eye while at the same time reversing the image in the mirror at the end of the box, allowed him to confuse the brain into thinking that in fact the man was opening his right hand; the hand that didn't exist, but the place from where came his phantom limb pain. A number of sessions that would last half an hour or so of repetition of closing the eye and hand and then opening again, eventually allowed the brain to agree that in fact the man did have a right arm. This in turn allowed the man's feed-back loop system to send the message back to the brain telling it that the hand had opened, which consequentially took away the pain of the fingernails digging into the palm of the man's hand. All in all, quite a clever piece of brain engineering, that left the man pain-free.

An understanding of the origins of pain sensations and an ability to reduce or control pain levels have always been among the most important aspects of medical treatment. After all, it is usually pain that induces someone to seek treatment. Conditions that are not painful are typically ignored or tolerated. But an individual can feel pain in the uninjured part of the body when the pain actually originates in another part of the body. This phenomenon is called referred pain. Thus a person with pain in the two middle fingers can often be found to have a problem in their thoracic spine (between the shoulders). More often than not sciatic persistent pain in the back of the thigh, calf and foot is caused by pressure on a nerve in the lumbar spine (base of the back). It can be caused by pressure on the nerve as a result of a poor sitting posture or in a badly designed seat.

Some days I dreamed of being pain free. Perchance the theory was that I should give in and accept the inevitable. Have some months off work, visit an orthopaedic surgeon and perhaps after a bit of surgery he would have wheeled me out as an invalid.

With a blue disabled persons disk on my car windscreen gosh, I could park wherever I cared without the least risk of a parking ticket. But no! This was not the answer. Work came first. I had a mortgage to pay and with children to support through university it gave me the need to work hard. I had no choice. I just had to accept the pain and get on with life, no matter how hard it could be at times.

Chapter Five

MARRIAGE

I am today still happily married to the same woman who joined me at the altar all of 34 years ago. Not all of it has been as sweet as it could have been. I admit I caused most of the problems. My excuse is that men are not good at marriage. We are simply not given the lessons on how to do it properly. Women cling to their mothers coat-tails. Men – me, well I just went my own way. I didn't have any time to listen to my mother in my youthful days. I was more interested in enjoying myself and, dashing around trying to make a shilling wherever I could.

Today, I accept that I was a lucky man to find the woman who agreed to take me as her husband. Despite all of the trials and tribulations, Sheila and I have raised two lovely children. We have made this marriage a success by working at it together. Well, perhaps I should admit that she worked at keeping it together when many a time it could easily have fragmented under the avalanche of trauma that I brought it from time to time. Now older and much wiser I am thankful that, despite all of the ups and downs, we love each other dearly. There are no instruction manuals or school lessons and yet most of us make a marriage survive, in one way or another. The subject of my next book, perhaps!

In the course of this marriage my back had to carry much of the burden. Like many newly married couples we were poor in the early days of our marriage, not that we are rich now! I trained as a quantity surveyor in the construction industry. Being an inquisitive sort of chap I worked hard to learn the many aspects of house building. In an effort to give us some quality of life and to keep costs to the minimum, I completed most of the construction work required in each of the houses that we lived in.

My woodworking skills learned at school are pretty good and thus I manufactured a lot of the furniture for the houses. Indeed we still have some of it today.

The first two houses were conversions of existing old property. The third house was built from scratch. It was hard work digging

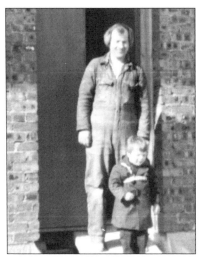

James Steele with son (Anthony), at the door of the new house under construction.

and concreting the foundations. Mixing the plaster, putting it on the wall and all of the other manual chores necessary to turn a pile of bricks, timber, roof slates and such into something that would shelter my new family was a strain on my puny skeletal frame.

I looked for little help in these toils and was happy to work mostly on my own. At times though, this did add to the strain on my muscles, ligaments and tendons. Lifting eight feet by four feet sheets of plasterboard, (2400mm x 1200mm for you metric buffs) staggering around with them on a scaffold as I held them above my head before fixing them to the ceiling, stretched my muscles to the limit. It was a bit of a balancing act as I took the weight of the whole sheet of plasterboard on my head while I positioned it with one hand and nailed it to the framing with the other. The pressure on my skeletal system and joints was huge.

I had to lock the board in position as I struggled to find the spot to fix the first nail. I used the top of my head to jam the board in place as I did this. To protect the thin muscles, the skin and the hair on the top of my head I would wear a woolly hat. In those days I had a good head of hair but today I am follically challenged. It is more than likely that a lot of it rubbed off, when I was making great effort nailing the plasterboard. However, I can see no link between bad backs and loss of hair! The tough grind of the construction work kept me fit, but I can remember many nights when I went home after working on our house feeling pretty stiff and sore. In those days a hot bath usually alleviated at least some of the aches and pains. Sadly it did nothing for hair retention.

The work I did in building and renovating the houses in which we have lived was painful. What it did by way of damage to my back in the long term I have no knowledge. If I had known better I would have started each work phase with a warm up. However, I was at that time unaware of the benefit of this simple form of protective exercise.

There are though other matters in marriage that possibly hurt my back. Raising a family eventually meant that my children, as they grew, came to an age where they wanted me to carry them, rather than to be wheeled around in a pram. Bending forward and

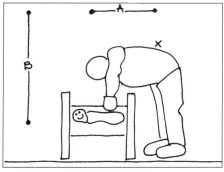

Sketch of man lifting child from cot (bent over it)

lifting them from the floor or from a cot was a stupid thing to do, but then I knew nothing about ergonomics.

Now a little older and hopefully more astute, let me share with you my wisdom.

The calculation of the pressure on point 'X' in the back is as follows:

(Weight of baby) x (distance A) x (height of lift B) = Kn of strain on the back.

When we walk, in theory we ought to do so standing vertically. Thus our centre of gravity should be through the middle of the body. In the sketch (above) the centre of gravity is in a downward motion through the middle of the baby and the person doing the lifting is much off balance. Thus the weight of the baby of say 30lb is converted to a point load on the back of approximately 180lb. Lifting a baby in this manner is a pretty stupid thing to do, but we all do it. I did it many a time. What I should have done was to bend my knees and keep my back straight when lifting the baby from the cot. Then I would have been using the strong muscles in my legs rather than testing the weaker muscles in my back. However, hindsight is great. Thus an appropriate and sensible chapter on lifting is something that I have given some words to later in the book. I would urge you to read carefully. It might just make the difference between a normal life and one afflicted with back pain.

But marriage put a strain on my back in other ways. Cooking for the family was an example. How could this be you may ask? Well, I married my wife for attributes other than her cooking ability. I am fond of good eating and so we agreed long ago that I would take the task of producing our food on a daily basis. Now I have an extensive library of cookery books. In 1989, I competed in the final of the Scottish Super Cook, a competition for amateur chefs. But, as I have probably eaten more than my fair share of what I have cooked I have in consequence a belly that is fatter than it should be.

Women tend to put weight on around the hips. It is therefore much more evenly distributed, but in men the tummy muscles get slack and the weight (fat) builds on the front. For men this is not at all clever as the fat is over many of our most important organs.

I enjoy my food but it has made me the chubby person that I am today. This is despite the fact that I have always trimmed the fat from every bit of meat that I purchase. I cook with olive oil much as they do in the Mediterranean countries. Apparently it comes out from your body much as it goes in. As far as I know it does no harm to the arteries, but over-use will make you obese. Of course there are many tales about the healthy habits of the Mediterranean people and the theory that by following their type of diet you may have a chance of living longer: olive oil, fresh fruit and vegetables, red wine, etc. I am sure that although they live longer, the chances are that they have just as bad backs as we have.

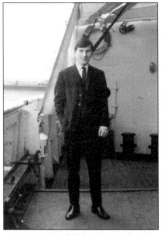

A young (and thin) James Steele on the M.V. "Irish Coast".

Everything in moderation, I think is the best advice I could give when it comes to food consumption. In my days as a student, working in the summer holiday from college, on the Belfast boat, I was a steady 147 pounds (67 kg). Even in the early days of marriage, I was the same weight.

Today, at 196 pounds (89kg), I am a little too heavy. The big problem is that at the age of fifty and a bit, it is difficult to lose weight without going on a diet of tasteless vegetables and such like. I have tried the diet of rabbit food (nothing but greens) and so on. It makes me extremely grumpy and probably hard to live with. I doubt that there are very few people out there who can begin a diet and stick to it. Women, for whatever reason, seem to be better at this than men. Perhaps they have more will-power.

Of course there will always be the exception to the rule, but a lot of us who have bad backs have them because we are overweight. The problem is exacerbated by the fact that the weight is mostly carried in the tummy region. The muscles struggle to cope with the additional weight they have to carry, with of course the consequent strain on the whole back. In a later chapter I will explain in more detail about the muscle structure in the body but as you can imagine the weight of the belly with the fat at the front is hardly good for us. Despite the fact that I am overweight I eat a healthy diet that contains all sorts of oily fish, wheat germ, fresh vegetables and so on; all of which is supposed to be good for us. It's just as I have said that I probably eat too much of it. Calories in - calories out and all that!

The over-consumption of alcohol is dangerous and can be a hazard to a marriage. It would be my opinion it was damaging to my back and a contributing factor to my pain and ills. You may think that I am mad to make such a statement, however I have good reason to come to this conclusion.

As my children grew up I needed somewhere to escape the daily household grind. Somewhere for a little manly relaxation! I found it first of all at the local political club, where they had four fine snooker tables. Bending over the green baize, I found to be good for my back. The gentle exercise seemed to massage the muscles. The intake of draft beer at the same time may have something to do with the easement, but I accept that it was probably the beginning of my beer-belly.

In those days my stomach muscles were strong. Rectus abdominus, external oblique, internal oblique and transverse abdominus are the muscles of the stomach that held me straight. They form a muscular girdle in an immense overlapping arrangement that helps to stabilise my entire abdominal region. Now I admit that I used and abused them. Later I became involved in the local rugby club. The hospitality of most rugby clubs goes without saying. Consuming copious amounts of beer after matches was the norm. After ten years on committee at Kilmarnock RFC I was appointed president. I was proud of the blazer awarded with this lofty position but not the belly that grew under it.

When we moved to Troon I gave up rugby and snooker. Now I spend a little time propping up the bar in my favourite local pub. Local is hardly the word to describe it in that it is three miles away. However, I have long since accepted that walking to the pub (and back) is a necessity. It has been proved without a shadow of a doubt, that everyday walking is good for back muscles. It keeps them in trim and at the same time looks after the heart.

The heart is affected by the movements of the diaphragm in that its pericardium (fibrous sheath of the heart) is attached to the diaphragm's central tendon by way of ligaments. The heart literally rides up and down on the diaphragm as you breathe. Walking makes you breathe a little more often and thus massage the heart.

I find it difficult to find the time for exercise (even walking to the pub). I live, as we all do, in this fast track world where we have mortgages to pay, deadlines to meet and so on. I could easily make excuses and never find the time to exercise, but these days I am a bit more ruthless and accept that it is a necessity. Many of us work hard, perhaps with a lot time spent behind the wheel of a motorcar. At the end of the day we arrive home, cook supper and then collapse in front of the television for the remainder of the evening. A good brisk walk before supper would make sense, but how many of us would contemplate it?

If you are lazy by nature and you don't do the sensible bit by exercising, then the advice that I can give at this point is to look at your posture. If you sit on a comfy sofa, don't slouch. Try to sit comfortably, with good support in the small of your back. If you are going through a period of back pain, then stuff all sorts of soft cushions behind you when you sit. Fill all of the gaps. This will encourage the muscles to relax and heal rather than allowing them to remain in a stiff and hurt condition.

Many people have terrible habits when they drive, spending most of the day peering over the steering wheel with all of the attendant muscle and joint strain that this causes. When I was younger I had a little car that had a bucket seat (as most cars did in those days), which did my back no good at all. It took me a long time to realise that when driving, you should have a comfortable position behind the wheel.

The seat position should be such that you don't stretch for the controls. The legs should be bent. I didn't have the money to purchase a car with good seating and thus I had to fit a rolled up towel, a cushion or some sort of lumbar support in the small of my back. Sheila who was my girlfriend was good at making something that could be more permanently fixed in the driver's seat as I have shown in the sketch under.

In sketch (A) there is inadequate lumbar support. This results in collapse of the chest forward, rounding of the shoulders and extension of the head again in a forward position. In sketch (B) the use of a lumbar support corrects this.

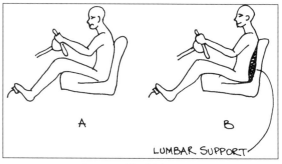

Posture while driving a car.

In the evening, at least after my supper has gone down, I always try to relax by reading the daily newspaper, or watching a bit of TV. A favourite position that I have is lying on the floor, face down, with my chin resting on my elbows, or with my arms folded under my chest. With my back curled in the opposite direction to what it has been in all day, I find this very therapeutic, as it tends to stretch all the ligaments and muscles, helping to take them back to the position that they should be in my back, rather than where they have been.

Sometimes I have to accompany my wife to the local supermarket. If you have to do this, (voluntarily or otherwise) give a thought to how you carry the bags of groceries. Two half filled bags (one on each hand) are better than one full bag dangling from one side of your body. Never load the bags such that they are a struggle to lift. In doing so there is a risk that the ligaments in the back may become distorted with the consequential threat of the muscles going into spasm. Hurt ligaments and muscles will hold themselves in the new position and the pelvis will as a result become tilted. I have done this often and ended up walking down the street like an old man, leaning to the side. So, use your head. There is more to hurt than your wallet when you shop.

Marriage though, has its positive side. The lady I cuddle up to at bedtime, especially on a cold winters evening, is a benefit. The good woman has been my rock in the worst of times and especially when I have been doubled up with back pain. I would have gone to the office many a morning in a dreadful physical state, if she had not bucked me up with a few well-chosen tender words. Feeling sorry for myself she was always on hand to help me dress. Simple things such as trying to bend to pull my trousers on were nigh impossible when I could not stoop because of muscle spasm. I have so much to thank her for and could not have managed without her.

Sheila helps with the garden. Well, actually she does all of the hard digging and lifting, planting and weeding. Indeed, all that it takes to keep the garden looking good. I just sit on my wee tractor going round in circles, cutting the grass and pretending that I am important. She had the logic to change all of the regularly used items in the kitchen from the bottom drawers to ones at a higher level. She often ties my shoelaces. This saves me the risk of hurting my back by bending in the morning, when of course it is not in its most supple state. What a sensible person she is and indeed what would I do without her?

If you are on your own, you will just have to devise all of your own tricks, to overcome the problems of dressing, lifting and bending and so on.

I laugh when I think of a business trip that I once made to the north of Scotland. I was just about to leave home and remembered that I had to take some sample bags with me. It must have been a good day in that I was pain-free. I drove my car round to my garage to where the bags were stored. With little regard to correct procedure I thoughtlessly lifted the bags into the boot of my car. I hurt my back, winced with pain and cursed! What a stupid clumsy person I was. I knew that the muscles would take some time to heal. This would be a simple matter if I could return to my house and take it easy for a few days. But, I had to embark on this important three-day business trip. A journey of about seven hundred miles lay ahead. I had little choice but to squeeze myself into the seat of my car, make myself as comfortable as possible and set off on this journey. Long hours behind the wheel are bad news if your back muscles are in spasm. I accepted that I would just have to grin and bear it and busied myself with the rigours of the journey.

Arriving at a hotel, in Inverness in the north of Scotland, I checked in. By now my back was extremely stiff and sore. I made my way to the room that had been allotted. Accepting that I had to do something to ease my pain and unwilling to succumb to yet more horrible pain-killers that I knew just burned a hole in my stomach, I attempted some of the emergency exercises I knew at that time. My back eased a little. After a meal I gingerly prepared for bed. Getting undressed at night is not too bad, as I could virtually undo my clothes, allow them to drop to the floor and step out of them. In the morning I knew that it would be a totally different matter. Especially when I would be on my own with no wife to help me!

I slept fitfully and woke at dawn. There was little sense staying in bed. In any case I had a job to do. I dressed carefully, taking steps wherever possible to ensure that I did nothing to unsettle my fragile back muscles. I managed most of the clothes but accepted that bending to attempt to put my socks on was stupid and downright dangerous. I just had to acknowledge the fact that I would have to spend the day without them.

One of the girls who had the job of cleaning the hotel rooms was setting up her trolley to start her morning round. Her closet was next to my bedroom. I had a little bit of a brain-wave. Taking my courage in both hands I asked the girl if she could put my socks on. To my amazement she readily agreed. When she was down at my feet, I felt like Jesus having his feet washed. I was so humble that the girl had agreed to my request. I was shocked though, when she told me that this was not the first time that she had been asked to do such a thing. More business men than care to admit, it would seem, have muscle spasm and suffer as I did. I was so grateful to the girl for her kindness. As I am sure were all of the fellows before me who had asked for the same assistance.

It was a good job my socks were clean! It reminded me of my mother who insisted on clean underwear every day, just in case she had an accident and ended up in the casualty department at the local hospital.

The event in the hotel was the final bit in the jigsaw, which convinced me that I should waste no time in writing this book. There must be a lot of us out there suffering in silence with little advice on how to manage back pain. Of course if you have had the

44

sense to purchase this book then you may acquire more than a few tips on how to handle the things that at times really get you down.

So there you have it, some of the good bits and the bad bits of marriage and how it affected my back. Had I been single, I'm sure that I would have been in a frantic state many a time, with no one there to help me. Fortunately, I wed a good woman who had the wisdom and understanding far beyond anything I could offer the marriage, especially in its early days.

Chapter Six

SEX (with a bad back)

I fully expect that most of the people who have purchased this book have bought it for practical advice about back pain and anticipate that the words written will be in an impersonal and clinical way.

However, back pain is something that afflicts not just older people, but young folk just as well, and allowing that mankind can be replicated, on the whole it is the young who will be doing the replicating. When we are young and have the desire to get on with what God planned, it can be a difficult and painful experience for those suffering with back pain. Thus I thought that it would make sense to write some words about the problems that I had to face at this time of my life.

I have no wish to offend anyone who reads this book. However, it is my opinion that this chapter as written has, for a number of reasons, a place in the book. If you feel that reading this may offend in any way, then please skip to the next chapter.

When I was a lad, the boys got the blame whenever an un-expected pregnancy materialised. Yet today it appears that the girls probably want to have full-blown sex as much as the boys. I don't see much self-restraint. Of course it is unfair of me to be making such a comment especially as I am now an old fuddy-duddy, eulogising about the pro's and con's and the do's and don'ts of what the young people of today should be up to, when in actual fact it has nothing to do with me. Nonetheless, the sexual act between a man and a woman is necessary in the creation of children.

As for my own sexual experiences I have been lucky. Sheila is my beautiful wife. This lovely woman (or the girl as she was then) helped me to find my way through these secret things. Sweet as apple cider, she was sensible, yet gentle, affectionate and caring in the development of our relationship. In the days before free sex for all, we respected the teachings of our parents, the pleadings of the Church and so on. Life did not revolve around sex, as sadly it does seem to do today. Thus we were content to take time with things. Beginning with kissing and cuddling, we discovered each other gradually. We were content. Sheila is very level-headed. The anchor in my life, I hardly appreciated it at the time. Now many years down the line, I can understand what a lucky man I am to have had such a dependable woman who has been the stabiliser in our marriage in more matters than our sexual relationship.

When our relationship was new and we were still finding out about each other, no matter how much or how little we kissed and cuddled, we always enjoyed it. The bond between us developed and then we married. In the years since, our sex life has gradually developed. It is an important part of our happy and stable marriage. In this joyful existence we got into the habit of having a pleasurable experience. Thus many a cold winter night in our early-married days was warmed by a joyous coming together. However in the midst of this and as the years went by my back pain evolved. My libido was not affected and despite my weakening back and the risk of un-expected painful muscle spasm the desire to make love to the beautiful woman I lived with remained strong.

I can remember more that one evening when in the middle of a lovely event I would suddenly be afflicted with muscle paroxysm. My back muscles would shudder. I would sweat with the pain. My body would scream at me to stop, yet my brain would urge me on to the pleasurable climax that I yearned. I found it impossible to explain to the woman I was sharing this loving with that the very act was hurting me.

The fact that I knew that she enjoyed our love making as much as I did, simply exacerbated the situation.

In those days I was convinced that men who are athletic were surely what all women looked for. I was worried that I did not fit into this category and that my back problem would affect our relationship. I didn't have the pluck to tell her that I had a problem. No matter how hard I tried I just could not get the words out. I became anxious that she would hate me for being such a failure.

Back pain of course can manifest itself in many ways that can affect a marriage. It does not necessarily have to happen in the midst of a sexual encounter. Every young man should be able to provide for his family. However, in the early days of our married life, money was tight and we had to make savings wherever we could. Thus digging the garden and cultivating fresh food to feed my children, was an important part of life. Attempting to lift big clods of soil in the midst of this work was dangerous for someone like me, with a weak back. However I had my pride, and no matter the risk, I could not allow my wife to attempt such a manual task, and had to do it all myself. The gardening work that I really shouldn't have attempted allowed often that I had to make an excuse and give up with the task far from complete. Simply stated, my back just wouldn't take any more punishment and I knew that excruciating muscle spasm would result if I continued with such a chore.

I was though often reluctant to give in to the pain but being at that time a belligerent Scotsman, despite the ache I often just wouldn't give in. To allow things to heal and to let the pain subside I spent many a time lying flat on the floor. Rest was the only thing that I knew at the time to help. I knew of nothing else, but neither did my doctor, apart that was from the hot baths and pain killers that he would often prescribe.

Hurting my back with the hard work in the garden I could accept, but never did I consider that there was a risk of back pain when having sex. It was not in any manual. The first time that it happened it was a shock. In addition to the pain, I was as explained, mortified. Allowing that I couldn't enlighten the woman that I lived with of my problem, I would never have been able to find the words to explain the scenario to my doctor. I suppose it was one of those things like bed-wetting that families keep a secret. Thus my back pain during lovemaking was a secret, for a long time. I suppose that Sheila despite my lack of words on the subject eventually worked out that all was not well. Ultimately and probably after a bit of cajoling I confided my problem. Thus together we worked out ways to enjoy our sex life without endangering my fragile back.

But other people have similar problems.

A woman I was acquainted with confided with me. She knew that I was afflicted with back pain. She told me that she had seen me suffer and that she had as I did a bad back. She was the wife of a famous athlete. He was one of the greats, something that Scotland produces just once in a while. She was a good-looking woman, indeed one to be desired, but in her mind she was nothing when compared to the star that shared her life.

Both she and her husband were our friends. Of course she never discussed her sex life. Nonetheless, Sheila and I met with them socially and would often enjoy the good food that we would share on a Saturday evening. At one such dinner party and perhaps with more alcohol in her blood stream than was good for her she told me that her bad back was a problem when she made love to her lovely husband. She had to hold back her emotions. A full-blown orgasm, she said would have been just too much for her back muscles to take. I was a bit puzzled at the time and surprised that she told me her secret.

Why she had to hold back her orgasm, when, my goodness, she did want to have one, was simply that her back muscles went into spasm if she had one. Thus she had to restrain herself in her lovemaking. The orgasm would be good, yet the consequential painful muscle spasm that would undoubtedly follow, wasn't worth the pain. Prior to hearing this story it had never crossed my mind that such a thing could happen to a woman. Back pain is a man thing, I thought. Of course now I know better.

Having overcome the problem with my back pain in the bedroom I still had simple daily tasks to complete. Dressing, at times was difficult and especially so in tying shoe-laces and such, but in my times of need my sympathetic partner was critical to my survival. I was a proud man, but had to bite-the-bullet, swallow my pride and ask for her help. Life has to go on. Hence I am eternally grateful to have had the wonderful Sheila to have helped me many a day with these menial tasks. These everyday tasks are nothing to a fit person, but completing these ordinary jobs meant so much to someone who suffers as I did with terrible and debilitating back pain.

Impromptu sexual events of course are difficult to cater for, but if you follow a few simple guidelines, even these situations can be coped with. Both young men and women will find it difficult to admit to a partner, that the act of love making, is something which although having a willing mind, the body will be weak. However, assuming that your partner has been with you for a while, not just a one night stand, he or she will be with you for more than what can be achieved under the bed clothes.

Accepting that many of us have back pain it is still possible to have a reasonably respectable sex life, simply by cuddling in an intimate manner. Stroking a partner in the erogenous zones can be extremely fulfilling. The full sexual act is not always necessary.

Snuggling together in a warm embrace, kissing fondly, can be at times most fulfilling and it won't do much damage to the back. I could not possibly advise on the love making position for a woman with a bad back, but the principles suggested, are much the same for both sides.

The erogenous zones, the areas that include the genitals, breasts and mouth are sensitive to touch and stimulation. They can be aroused as you lie beside your partner, with no danger to someone with a bad back, but every chance of creative interplay. It is possible to drive a lover up the wall simply by skilfully lightly touching and caressing various parts of the body. Touching around the erectile tissue of the breasts leads to a high pitch of anticipation for the fondling of the nipple itself.

The secret in the success of this type of lovemaking is to keep your lover in the dark about what your next move will be. Gently caressing the breast and surrounding chest can be followed by suddenly addressing the nipple, tenderly squeezing it between the fingers, then just as your partner is experiencing their pleasure the fingers move away to stroke another part of the body. Then just as suddenly as you left the nipple, return to it. Repeating this process can be particularly sexually stimulating. Of course, it is possible to replace the fingers with the tongue to enhance the experience.

Nipples addressed in this manner become hard and stimulate erotic feelings in other parts of the body. Of course the genital area can and will be where your partner will expect you to gravitate. However the secret is to take things slowly. Start with soft strokes of the tummy, knees, and inner thigh, avoiding any contact with the sex organs. This will heighten the emotion and desire of your lover. Lightly flitting from one part of the body to the other but generally around the genital area will arouse and excite. Your partner will not know where you are going to touch next.

However we can all handle just so much stimulation and eventually the genital organs will have to be stroked, with your partner demanding an orgasm break.

The mouth has a big part to play in any sex act. The lips impart the kiss of sex. They are evocative. All body parts enjoy the soft wet sensations of mouth play. It is a giver as well as a receiver. Of course this leads us to oral sex. (My old English schoolteacher will be turning in her grave, at the thought of me writing about a subject such as this!) This is something that would appear to form part of a relationship in its first blush. Something that younger people will indulge in more readily. The odd occasion when it may happen, in a longer term relationship really needs something special to make it spark. However, again it is a form of sex, which will hardly test the structure of the back.

In a stable relationship, where both of you love each other intensely, it should be possible to complete some rather fulfilling oral sex, assuming that is that you have a sympathetic partner. In a man, there is no need to be ashamed to admit that extremely active sex could leave you in a painful situation. However surmising that most of us reading this book might be a bit beyond the first flush of youth, oral sex might just be a little out of the question.

And so to fulfil the needs of the both partners, we have to find some other method. Virtually the entire skin surface responds well to feathery touches. As a result, I have found that my sex life is now safe and free from the risk of back pain. At the same time my wife as far as I can gather is happy with what I have to offer, indeed simply wrapping in a warm embrace, and hugging is pleasurable.

Not all sex has to be in the bedroom. Many a happy hour can be spent in the bath. The bathroom should be warm, scented and candle lit. Full-blown sex is not necessary. Simple water sports can have many forms. Take turns to wash each other's bodies from head to toe and take time to do a thorough sensitive rinsing job before towelling each other dry. A warm milky drink and both of you will be ready for whatever comes later in the bedroom.

This may take the form of massage. Not many of us are trained in the art. Nevertheless, most of us have some kind of idea. It is an effective drugless therapy. Using a good quality fragrant oil helps. There are few parts of the body that don't benefit from it. In the process the circulation is enhanced and skin and muscle tone can be improved. The real bonus is an overall feeling of well-being. It soothes, stimulates and is often the precursor to foreplay.

A truly professional massage is involved and takes time to learn. There are many movements and intricacies required for a quality full body rub down. However, for those of us without the qualifications the secret is light touch. Simply stated, don't rub hard. The last thing your partner wants is somebody trying to squash the living daylights out of them. Be gentle. It will pay dividends. Massage serves to soothe the skin and nerves. It relaxes the muscles and calms the mind. There are no set movements. Just do what feels right for you and your partner and make sure that you move in smooth motions. My wife is adept at this simple form. Often at the end of a stressful day she has helped me drift off into a comfortable and restful sleep.

We have thus worked out ways to enjoy our sex life without endangering my back. Of course I can remember when jumping off the wardrobe was the norm. However, then I went through the whole spectrum of ever increasing back pain. It is true to say that there were many times when I was not interested in sex as my back pain consumed all. However as I came to terms with it, my libido returned.

The main requirement for good sex is that you both have to be fulfilled. How you reach this happy and contented state is for each partner to be willing to satisfy the other in the way he/she likes best. From a male point of view I have found that female responses to sex are more complex than the male's. Subtler sensitive touching thankfully gratifies women! Accepting and recognising this, we have had the perfect marriage of sex and cuddling, giving and receiving.

In the broader terms it is important if you have a bad back to think about what you can do to prevent a difficult situation. I can't see any books written about the subject, and additionally I am no expert. Perhaps though from some of my exercises you may glean some information from the gentle warm-ups (psoas, knee lifts etc) that may help prevent a catastrophe. As a last resort send me an e-mail through my web site www.bnth.org if you have a query.

Chapter Seven

MY PHANTOM ULCER

In my early married life I worked as a quantity surveyor for a construction company. The hours were long but I had the need to earn hard cash to support my little family and pay the mortgage on our new home. One dwelling was a modest red sandstone terraced house, near to the primary school our children attended and adjacent to a park where they played in evenings. It was our pride and joy.

The house required an awful lot of work to bring it up to a tolerable standard. With little cash to spare, I had no option but to do the work myself. I fitted a warm air central heating system, rewired the electrics, constructed a new bathroom and painted and decorated as necessary. Our new kitchen was converted from the old washhouse. The consequential strain and back pain resulting from all of this effort was considerable.

We lived in the house for three years and in that time turned a handsome profit on our investment. This gave us the financial ability to think about building a new home. And so we looked for a plot of land where our dream could be realised. Land was difficult to find. However one day the local Council advertised the sale of a bit of land in the best part of the town.

Most plots of land in those days, on which a house could be built, were sold for something in the region of £3,000. Allowing though that there had been few, if any, plots sold in the town for some years we knew that it would not sell cheaply. We took some advice and offered three times the price. It seemed a mad thing to do, but in actual fact we won it by just a few pounds. In time it was to prove a very wise investment.

Thus I set about designing a home for our family and prepared my estimate for the cost of the construction. I accepted that as I had many of the necessary skills that I would just have to do a lot of the back breaking work on my own, but nothing is cheaper than your own labour.

The stress of having to work during the day for my employer and then work at nights and weekends on the building work of the new house, took its toll. I was burning the candle at both ends. When you are young this does not seem to matter so much as the body is able to regenerate and recover much quicker. However, eventually we decided that we just had to have a holiday. It was to be the first we had had since we married. A package trip to the island of Majorca was organised.

We set off from Glasgow airport. It was the first time our 3 year old daughter Deborah had been on an aeroplane. I still smile when I think of her asking why the picture on the window was moving as we took off. Indeed, it was the first time that my wife had flown, never mind my daughter. We settled in a resort hotel. It had a reputation for good food. In the evenings though, it was very quiet and had little in the way of entertainment. It was our first ever experience of life in a warm climate and it was a strange feeling living in a hotel, which had no carpets on the floor. Polished granite and marble were the norm.

On return from holiday, I had a pain in my tummy that just would not go away. I suffered for a week or two and then succumbed to a visit to the doctor. I was proud that I was a rare visitor to his surgery. I could not remember the last time I paid him a visit. I had the constitution of an ox. Yet now for the first time in years I was ill with stomach pain.

The doctor was an elderly gentleman. He lived in a big house in the best street in town and he drove a Rolls Royce. Not bad for a family practitioner! The trappings did not improve his doctoral skills, as I was to find to my regret. He had a prod at my tummy and agreeing with him that it did hurt where he was pressing, he declared that I had the beginnings of an ulcer.

I had always taken the attitude that if the locals can eat it, then so can I. Thus on holiday I had consumed the squid, the octopus, and the wild boar. Indeed anything that was offered. It wasn't going to hurt me! A tough man from Scotland, having the stomach of an ox, I could eat steel girders! As you can imagine it was a surprise therefore to be told that I had an ulcer. But I had to believe a man with such a wealth of medical knowledge. My doctor was beyond reproach, or so I thought. As it was to show in time I was a fool to believe him!

Then followed months when I must have consumed every kind of stomach sedative. Gone were the days when I could consume portions of my favourite fried fish and chips. Pints of beer at my local rugby club were simply out of the question. Just little bits of these types of food or drinks gave me excruciating soreness. My stomach muscles would spasm and I would be left writhing in pain.

As you can imagine my eating habits changed dramatically.

In consequence I became thinner. My back pain came and went. It seemed to go through from the tummy to the spine. Then being the silly person that I was at the time, stupid thoughts came to mind. Did I have cancer? Was I going to die? Lord, I had all sorts of dreams about the bad things that I thought were happening to me. Now I was a regular at the doctor's surgery. My medical history file began to fill with alarming alacrity.

This horrible life style was now the norm. Looking back, I must have been grumpy and pretty hard to live with. I don't know how Sheila or the children put up with me. However they made little of my bad tempered ways. In a way, I suppose that they just let me get on with it. I must have been hard to live with.

On one of my regular visits I found that my old doctor had retired and left me in the hands of a young newly qualified doctor. I wondered what indeed this new fellow would know about my medical history and the problems that I had with my ulcers. I don't know why but I didn't trust him. Thus our meetings were an ever-narrowing path of collision. I was convinced that this upstart knew nothing. He was no doubt convinced that I was an idiotic troublesome patient.

At the previously mentioned political club, where I enjoyed a game of snooker, I was reduced to quaffing milk stout. My stomach just would not accept anything stronger. Quite a few of the older chaps in the club had had or were suffering from ulcers of one kind or the other. They made it obvious that my new young doctor was trying to save the funds of the Health Service, by refusing to prescribe the expensive tablets, which were sure to solve my problem. Dispensed in the amounts I demanded would probably bankrupt his practice. But what did I care. My new doctor and I were at loggerheads.

Eventually we had words. I threatened to report him to the medical profession for incompetence. How could such an inexperienced fellow have any idea what was wrong with me? Exactly what kind of game was he playing with my health? Why was he refusing to prescribe the strong stomach pills I so obviously needed? The lads at the snooker table had to be right! Eventually he gave in and prescribed what I had been demanding for months.

What care had I to the cost to the nation! I was ill. I deserved this medication, just as much as any other unfortunate. And so I thought that this would be the end of my troubles. The pain in the tummy and the mirrored pain in the low back would soon be gone.

Sadly, despite consuming his boxes of expensive pills I was no better. Soon it was back to his office for another confrontation. The stupid man, could he not work out what was wrong with me?

After some discussion the doctor suggested that he would make an appointment for me at the local hospital. There they would carry out an endoscopy. Simply described, I would be taken into an operating theatre and after administering some anaesthetic they would slide a tube containing a TV camera down my throat. The surgeon could then have a look around my stomach to find the exact location of the ulcer.

In those days the unions had been at loggerheads with the government of the day. Strikes were the norm. In the week preceding the date of my admission to hospital the nurses were on strike. Run of the mill operations had all been cancelled.

I am not a stupid person but for whatever reason, I never imagined that nurses would strike. I was not aware that they had. Thus I turned up at the hospital at the prescribed time on the appointed date. It was strangely quiet.

Just by luck, the strike had been settled the previous day. The hospital having cancelled all non-essential operations had not one patient to fill their six operating theatres. To my amazement the nurse at reception had a hurried discussion with senior staff. It was agreed that they would admit me into the Day Surgery Unit.

What I did not know at the time was that I was to be wheeled into the teaching theatre, where I would have fifty or so prospective doctors and nurses watching the on goings through the glass above the operating table.

Prior to entering the theatre in an anti-room I undressed and put on one of those stupid green gowns, which tie up the back, but hardly hide your modesty. A fellow came in and asked me to climb onto a trolley. He covered my modesty with a white sheet. Thus attired he wheeled me into the pre-theatre room where a lovely nurse gave me an injection in the back of my hand. It made me feel a bit woozy, but not so that I was unconscious. After a while I was wheeled into theatre.

My first time ever in such a room, I was petrified. Especially so when I glanced up to see all of the expectant faces behind the glass! The fear of the unknown was my only concern. What indeed would these nasty doctors do to me? Would it hurt? Would they find me full of horrible ulcers? Would I be sick? Was I going to die? Did I have cancer? More importantly would I make a fool of myself in front of all of these young folk? Oh God why did you do this to me? Am I such a bad person? All sorts of nonsense whirred though my brain. Much of it repeated oft-times over!

I was asked to lie on my side. The nurse holding my hand tried her best to calm me. I looked over at a machine with all sorts of pipes and tubes emanating from it. They were all pretty thin. I thought to myself that I could after all probably swallow one of them, if that was what I had to do. The surgeon introduced himself. He described what he would attempt to do. I was shocked when he picked up a tube from the back of the machine. I had not seen it. It was as big as a hosepipe. How on earth did he expect me to swallow such a monstrous thing?

However, I did what I was told and started to swallow the tube. I choked. The nurse and the surgeon tried to make me relax. I felt as if I was about to vomit. They encouraged me as best they could and eventually the hose started to disappear. It seemed that they were pushing miles of the thing inside me. My eyes were filled with tears. The trainee doctors and nurses must have been having quite a chuckle at my uncomfortable squirming. I have had many a good battering on the rugby field, with never a word spoken. But on this table I was just a big coward.

Once the tube was in place the surgeon started to fiddle with the dials on the instrument panel. It was a remote control camera with an attached light, which could crawl around in my innards looking for my ulcer. After what seemed an eternity the tube was removed. I was wiped clean and wheeled to the recovery ward. I was shattered by the experience. I think that I slept for two or three hours.

Recovered from the effects of the anaesthetic, I was given some nourishment. I was starved, having had nothing to eat since the previous evening. Discussing the affair with the nurse looking after me I was relating the horrific event that I had just undertaken. She was understanding and listened to my tale, but probably had heard it all a hundred times before.

Just then the surgeon came into the room. He told me that he could find no ulcer. I had as good a set of insides as he had seen in a long time! I wondered why he could give me this kind of news. I knew that I had an ulcer. Could the stupid man not find it? We discussed the issue for a while. Eventually he left the room with the protests of an unhappy patient ringing in his ears. Later, I left the hospital with a sealed envelope, to be handed in at my doctor. I was hurt and angry.

The next day I made an appointment to see my young upstart doctor. I gave him the brown envelope. He opened it and read the words. There was not a trace of emotion on his face. I had no idea what had been written. I mumbled that they could not find the ulcer, but reminded him that there was no doubt that I had one.

He sighed deeply, laid the letter on the table and looked at me. Then he gave me the news that there was now just one last thing that he could do. He made an appointment for me to see another specialist.

The next week I presented myself at the hospital once again. The lady at reception indicated the direction of room 13/5. Was it to be my date with destiny?

Arriving at the door I looked up to see the words – Psychiatry. I knocked and entered. A friendly middle-aged well dressed gentleman greeted me. He asked me to sit. In the few minutes it had taken me to come into his room, my brain had been whirring as if it was working out a complicated mathematical equation. Suddenly it gave me the answer. It all clicked into place. I had worked out in my own head what was wrong with me.

NOTHING!

The brainless old doctor who months ago prodded my midriff and suggested that I had an ulcer had sown the seed. I was so stupid to believe him. Lord, did I feel brainless. Before the psychiatrist had time to commence his explanation, I blurted out that I was sorry to have wasted not just his time but also that of all of the hospital staff. Briefly I explained what I had just experienced. I was on my feet and out of the hospital at the speed of light.

Arriving home, I explained to my long-suffering wife what had happened. I apologised for all that I had put her through. I was sorry for the months of misery I had given her. I enlightened her about the silly old doctor convincing me that I had an ulcer. Within days, I was drinking pints of beer and having fried fish and chips for supper. All the taboos were gone. At the same time my back pain improved. It had all been in my head.

Chapter Seven

A STUPID PERSON

I cannot remember the first time that I injured my back. It seems such a long time ago. In addition to all of the other jobs that I have had in my life, as a lad I worked in the fertile potato fields on a farm near West Kilbride, about four miles from where I lived in Ardrossan. It was very hard back-breaking work. Yet, as I was driven home at the end of the working day, in the back of the tractor, I looked at the other young fellows who had as I had, toiled all day. I could not see the pained expression on their faces that I surely had on mine. I didn't have a clue as to why my back hurt and theirs didn't.

The various jobs that I had as a youth didn't help. At times they gave me pain. But, in youth I accepted the pain as part of my existence. Then I had other things in my life that took priority. Later in life, having to lift heavy sample bags in my daily work for a company that traded in the construction industry certainly had something to do with it. I was in my forties at the time. I did need the job and probably just accepted that lifting such bags in and out of the boot of my car as I visited various customers were part of my job. Knowing what I know now I could not have been more stupid. My employer gave no advice on how to or, more to the point, how not to lift these heavy samples.

When I was a lad, in common with all school kids I walked to school and then back home at the end of the day. I lived four miles from my somewhat stern institute. It was a hard struggle through the cold and often very wet Scottish winter weather. But returned from this place of learning and after tea we would play football for hours, no matter the weather conditions. Bad backs were something that did not exist. I wasn't bright but far from stupid. I was a healthy specimen.

Please don't get angry at me for getting on my high-horse; however it seems that much of what we stack up health-wise in later life will be a result of what sort of life we lead in childhood. Thus, I think that it is important that I am allowed to get on my soapbox, (just for a little while).

Fat kids will eventually lead to fat adults, many of whom will have a risk of back pain. A recent case study has suggested that one in four children in Scotland show signs of heart disease by the age of fourteen. The findings have been described as "frightening" and blame the fast food and computer game lifestyle now common in most children. Apparently the levels of cholesterol and sugar in 25% of the children tested were equivalent to results which would be considered as heart disease risk in adults. The sedentary life style of today's young people must be stacking up problems for themselves in later life and thus it comes as no surprise that the research has indicated that some parents may outlive their children.

Doctors are especially worried, as health problems are known to increase in adulthood, a simple result of the fact that too many of today's children are obese. Hamburger, chips and milkshake were hardly the type of food I ate as a child, yet this is the sorry mess that too many youngsters enjoy as a staple diet. How many of them walk to school? How stupid are they to put their own health at risk? What cares have they for a decent healthy diet? It makes me angry that parents allow it to happen. But then again, perhaps it is the parents who are to blame.

My parents were not silly people. They made sure that I ate none of the nonsense that young folk today seem to survive on. As a child, I can remember the horse and cart that came up the street and stopped at our front door every other day of the week. An old fashioned travelling shop, it sold fresh fish from the clean waters off the west coast of Scotland, and vegetables garnered from the local fields.

Thus many a day we would dine on herring or mackerel and potatoes. Good old-fashioned bony fish. Not pretty, but fine tasting and packed full of the right type of polyunsaturated fats. The type of fat found also in sunflower oil, rapeseed oil and Soya. Not that I was aware of this as a child. Today there is a leaning towards the monounsaturated fats that you will find in olive oil, hemp oil, peanuts and avocado. Apparently they are more able to cope with controlling our cholesterol levels, but as I say, as a child my diet was not that of the children of today. In addition I exercised regularly. Thus I was thin and healthy. My back pain may well be a genetic problem that I was born with. An unfortunate quirk of fate, it is one of those things that happen from time to time. I lived with it, accepted and got on with it. In time, it dragged me down and made me sad, bad and angry. However as you can see I have survived out the other side of it. I accept that I am not a perfect specimen these days, despite the fact that I do try to lead a healthy life. Thanks to the wisdom of my parents I didn't lead the unhealthy life that many of today's youngsters.

Many of the professional football teams in Scotland in those days were composed of lads who were Scottish. There were few, if any, players from overseas. The South African Johnny Hubbard who played for Glasgow Rangers, was one of the first to arrive on these shores.

Several of my more gifted pals strived to make it all the way in the football world. A few became quite famous and played for well respected teams. At the same time they earned a good salary. Sadly today many of our teams are composed of foreigners. Consequently the kids in the street don't play football. Indeed they seem to have a could-not-care-less attitude. Playing football has become a low priority. Many of them are fat and would much rather spend their time slumped on a sofa staring at a television. And so we have become a nation of football watchers rather than participants, much to the detriment of our national soccer team!

Hence I would have to ask how many of the back problems we have today are related to this "couch potato" syndrome. Too many of us just lie around at every opportunity, grazing on yet another calorie filled chocolate bar as we watch TV. Adding inches to the waistline, we are stacking up many health problems. The damage that will be done by reducing our ability to have muscles that are strong and supple enough to support our ever burgeoning frames is a worry. We cannot go on like this. So we must ask some questions.

How many of us exercise regularly? When was the last time you walked to collect some shopping and carried the filled bags all the way home? When did we last run up a flight of stairs? Cycle a bike? Spend some time in the swimming pool?

Getting out of breath is important. Everyone should have some form of daily exercise, which will make us breathe moderately heavily for at least thirty minutes. Exercise is not the drudge that many of us seem to think. Simple things such as those in the following list can make all the difference:

Use the stairs whenever you can.

Don't rely so much on the car. Park it five minutes from where you need to go shopping.

Take a 15 or 20 minute walk at lunch time.

Try doing a little housework or gardening every day.

Get off the bus one stop before your own and walk that little bit extra.

Remember that if you only exercise five minutes at a time, but do this six times a day, you've managed your daily 30 minutes of exercise. It's not ideal but it's better than nothing at all. The bonus in all of this is that people who exercise have a higher metabolic rate, so their bodies burn more kilojoules per minute, even when asleep.

Back in my childhood and teenage years exercise wasn't a chore; it was just part of life. Recreation was an every-day event. I spent my time running about playing football, or climbing trees to steal apples, and then being chased by a policeman: the local 'Bobby'. Even he was on foot.

Everyone walked somewhere, every day. Gosh, it had not been many years prior to the time that I started school, that kids went barefoot. The little money that the fathers earned in those days was just enough to buy food and heat the home. It did not stretch to footwear. I don't imagine that the barefoot children in Africa have back problems, nor indeed do they seem to have many of the Western health problems that have evolved with our lifestyle.

Accordingly as a lad I was not a stupid person. But with my changing life style as I grew up I did become one. By building and converting the various homes that we lived in, my back muscles were then probably stronger than they had ever been. In essence they were more able to support my frail skeletal frame than they are today. It was more likely that my problems evolved after I became a bit more financially successful in life. Then I began to pay others to do the manual jobs that I would normally have done myself. In other words, I got lazy. I was indeed a stupid person.

Fifteen years ago I was employed as a quantity surveyor, with a reputable and successful building company. My job was to measure the work done by the operatives at the various building sites under construction. I had to go to site, and climb the scaffolds erected around the buildings, where I would measure the work that was underway. This certainly got me out of breath. Indeed I was quite proud to be able to walk up six or more flights of stairs and at the same hold a conversation with the site manager who would normally be puffing to keep up.

One winter day at such a building site, I had climbed the scaffold ladders on a tall building under construction and was standing on some scaffold boards on the fourth floor level. The boards had been rain soaked the previous day and had become stiff, hard and slippery after a very cold and frosty Scottish winter night. Common sense would have called for some sand to sprinkle onto the greasy surface. But I was in a hurry. A stupid man! I attempted to do my measuring work and walk on this dangerous surface at the same time.

Of course I slipped. I did the splits. Both legs went in the opposite direction at the same time. My weak back could not take the strain. I screamed as I tore some muscle fibres, ligament or whatever at the base of my spine. Lord it hurt. But, I had a job to do. I had to complete my assignment, pain and all.

Finishing my work on the building site, I gingerly got into my car. Immobilising my back by settling into the well-supported seat I drove about thirty miles to the office. Arriving, I found that my back had stiffened and thus it was only with difficulty that could I extricate myself from the car. In the office someone said that I probably had a "slipped disk." Of course they knew as much about a slipped disk as I did. But in those days that was the common misconception of the problem.

The term 'slipped disc' is erroneous, as the disc is fixed in place. It could be better described as a herniated disk. The inescapable fact was that I had been a stupid person. The bother of going for a bucket of sand was just too much for the lazy person that I had become.

I don't intend to go into the medical terminology used to describe many of the problems with bad backs. Talking about circumferential tears that weaken the annulus and result in damage to the nucleus pulposis, is hardly what you want to read, no matter the extent of the diagrams attached. Thus I am trying to describe things in this little book in layman's terms.

So, let us return to another example of this "stupid person".

I have written a chapter about lifting and sitting, which explains how and what we should do to protect our backs in our daily life. Simple things that take the risk out of the equation! Yet in my early years I subjected my back to massive strain as I tried to manoeuvre various items necessary in the construction or renovation of the houses that we lived in. I suppose that I gave it little thought. I just worked through the pain, winced and got on with things. But as I was a stupid person I continued along the same path repeatedly damaging and, in consequence, weakening the same bit of my back.

The body has the ability to heal itself, but if you keep hurting the same spot, each time it takes a little bit longer to repair the problem. In time, it becomes just about impossible for things to heal. The body is worn out. The wear and tear might just become irreparable. Ergo my stupidity did revolve around hurting my back by lifting heavy things. However I also managed to hurt it in many other ways.

I am a lucky man and married as you are now aware to a smashing woman. A sensible person, she could see that I was struggling with my back problems and she encouraged me to try the local chiropractor to try and resolve my problem.

I had experimented with a variety of other so-called back cures. Thus I agreed to let my body be examined by this new form of repair mechanism that had recently arrived in Scotland. In the beginning it seemed to do the trick. My structural alignment improved. I must admit that I was afraid while the chiropractor carried out this strange form of manipulation. Crunching my body back into place hurt! A novice to this form of bizarre healing I took some convincing. However, in those days I knew of nothing else that gave my poor aching body any solace.

Thus for a while, I allowed my body to be manipulated in this manner, despite the frightening and perhaps dangerous positions that the therapist who manipulated my delicate body would get me into.

One morning, after an emergency visit to the chiropractor I returned to the workplace which my wife and I shared. By then I had my own little construction company and the office was our headquarters. It was a cosy little room, with just enough space for desks and shelves for the two of us. With my back seemingly repaired, my wife was pleased to see me. She kissed me tenderly. An amorous feeling began to percolate my brain as did a rising in my loins.

Despite the fact that at times I would be miserable with my back pain, my libido remained high. Allowing a bit of something that does one well at times seemed appropriate. And so some heavy petting with my good lady as we stood jammed against the wall, developed into something a bit more serious. Unfortunately, in the more steamy bits, with my mind racing, I forgot all about my back, never mind the activity it was being subjected to. And so, in the culmination of this particularly vigorous bit of lovemaking my back muscles gave out. The muscles around the ligaments in my lower back that I keep tearing went into spasm. I did not know whether to laugh or cry.

Eventually, I was calm. With less steam coming out of my ears, my wife helped me to recover from the painful muscle spasm. I struggled to the floor where I was able to complete the emergency back calming exercise that I knew at the time.

Later that evening we went to a party hosted by some good friends. My wife does not need a lot of alcohol to make her tipsy. She thought that it would be good to tell the tale of the events earlier in the day. So all at the party had a laugh at my expense! All in all, it described me as an amorous, but perhaps a brainless man!

The other times that I have been stupid and consequently hurt my back were mostly to do with playing golf as I will describe in the next chapter. Lifting heavy items though was the main cause of the pain that I suffered many a day.

Most of us when we hurt our backs don't really understand why it happens. Nor do we know the right type of therapy to help. This often leaves one in a very vulnerable situation, especially if you are a novice back pain sufferer and are not aware of the things that we can do to help ourselves, or the types of therapies that are available to repair the hurt to our backs. As a result I have been up many blind alleys looking for a 'cure'.

Taking some acupuncture may relieve the pain, but in my opinion it does not address the problem. I had treatment from a well-know fellow who has a clinic not far from where I live. After the first treatment I was of the opinion that it may be able to help me. However, after several visits to this man, I found that his treatment helped me less and less and so I stopped going. I do remember that at the end of every visit as I was about to leave his clinic The words "see you next week" would ring in my ears. At the time acupuncture was all that I knew that gave me some succour. I can see now that when you have patients that return week after week, that very soon you will become a rich man. Thankfully I got wise to this.

My visits to the chiropractor, I have to admit, lulled me into a false sense of security. It was new to the UK. There was just the one practitioner local to me. In the whole of the country I don't think that we had more than half a dozen. It was a strange therapy that people did not trust. Bone crunching - it makes me shiver when I think of what I allowed the therapist to do to me! Mr Crowbar they call it in the USA! Yet initially I was grateful when I found it. It was the only thing that gave me any relief from my back problems. It was my crutch. But just as with anything, if you abuse it, it will bite back.

The body needs time to heal in between treatments. I didn't give it any. After yet another visit to the chiropractor, I would be straight back to the golf course the next day. My back would survive the vagaries of a round of golf. I would convince myself that all was well. My back would stay fixed. Lulled into this false sense of security, I would, after a few days forget all about my pain! But being the stupid person I was I would lift something heavy or make a sudden awkward movement and do the damage all over again.

This would cause the cartilage (part of disc) to squeeze out of place and press the spinal nerve. The result invariably was shooting pain in my back and legs, often accompanied by numbness and tingling that I just didn't understand.

I knew that there must be a limit to the amount of manipulation that could be given to my, by now, ever weakening back, and was well aware that the only recourse to this perhaps irreparable damage may be to submit to the surgeon's knife. In those days surgery was invasive and involved a fairly large open incision, detaching muscle and ligament from bone. Now the same operation (known as endoscopic discectomy) is done through a small hole that requires no stitching when complete. However, I was a coward. Surgery was simply out of the question.

In the early part of married life (pre chiropractic) I can remember at times hurting my back quite severely. My first recourse would be to telephone the doctor. Invariably I was told to take some pain killers and sleep on the floor. At times I would subject myself to two or more nights at a time on the floor in the vain hope that I was helping things. What agony! Of course it did nothing to mend the hurt. Laying there in pain I would wonder what indeed doctors knew about back pain. I cursed them.

It seemed to me that the common resolve for doctors when dealing with back pain sufferers was to prescribe various pills. I often wondered if the doctors knew just what damage they were doing by allowing these mouthful's of analgesics to burn holes in the stomach of the poor unfortunate who was stuffing them down his throat. I came to the conclusion that doctors knew little about how to resolve back pain problems. All they did was to give a pill to mask the pain. Never did they offer anything that addressed the problem. My argument was reinforced when I read a back pain book written by an eminent professor from a University in Scotland. At great length he told about the structure of the back and all of the things that can go wrong with it. Yet, despite being a weighty tomb, not once did he give advice on how to resolve the problem.

Lying on your back for long periods is not good for it. I learned this from a physiotherapist who came to help me in an emergency one day. He was at the time the physiotherapist for the Scottish Football team and happened to live in the town where I resided. It was a Sunday when he came, not his normal day of work. I think that my wife must have been down on her hands and knees pleading when she asked him to come and help. I was in such pain. Home visits were not his sort of thing.

With his simple form of massage he was able to calm the

muscles in my back, which were in painful spasm. He advised that he could give no long-term cure and that I had to get to the root of the problem. He gave me advice on the firmness or otherwise of the bed that I slept on. He told me that if you lie on your back in bed and slide your hand under the small of your back you can test on the firmness, or otherwise of the mattress. Too easy to slide your hand under and the bed is too hard. The small of the back is not being supported. Difficult to slide your hand under and the bed is more than likely too soft. A halfway house between is the ideal solution. I am sure though that he looked upon me as being a bit stupid to get myself into the unhealthy state that I was.

On another occasion I went for treatment to a physiotherapist in Glasgow. I had to travel some thirty miles to get there. It was again at the weekend and sadly in this country although we have a fine health service, treating people with dodgy backs at the weekend is not on the priority list. Not one local therapist would take me as a patient on a Sunday. Thus I had to travel a distance to meet with this considerate woman. She was pretty decent and like most physiotherapists she knew her job. She told me that after six or seven attacks on the ligament, the scar tissue would be such that it would be more or less impossible to damage it. In other words, I should by now have stopped hurting it. Regrettably, I have not reached that stage yet where my back is not hurting, nor can I find any medical evidence to back up her claim. However, as you will find later in the book, I am making progress towards a pain free life.

I suppose that I could go on giving many examples of how I have been stupid. I think that what I am trying to counsel is that it is all in our own hands. I am sure that we could fill a book with the stupid things that we have all done. The sad thing is that despite the fact that we are all very aware that we are vulnerable, we still continue to be stupid.

We could and should take steps to prevent it. We only get one life. So it is important that we look after the body that God has given us. The problem is that we are all lazy. Rather than taking just a little exercise that will strengthen the back, we don't. We take risks putting our weak back in dangerous situations that invariably result in yet another round of painful muscle spasm. I am sure that my wife tired of having to come to my aid every time that I hurt myself, particularly when I did something stupid.

Our lives and the qualities that it has or doesn't have are in our own hands. So my advice would be to get off your butt and do something about it now. Don't waste another minute. Put this book down. Get some paper and a pen. Have a good think about what you do on a daily basis and write it down. Agree that a good bit of regular exercise might just be the tonic that your back muscles are crying out for. Never mind the benefit to the cardiovascular system. Change your life today. Then perhaps you won't be the stupid person that I was.

Chapter Nine

GOLF

At the age of sixteen or so I bashed some golf balls around the local municipal golf course. Armed with borrowed clubs, I was soon to have the bug and invested in a proper set. They were second hand but they were better than the hickory shafted clubs on loan from an uncle, (who taught me the basics in golf etiquette). Soon I became a reasonably good golfer. Today, I live in the small town of Troon, in the west of Scotland, where we are privileged to have six fine golf courses. It includes Royal Troon golf club, where the world watches when the Open Championship is played there every five or six years. In such a town, if you breathe and have legs then you must play golf. It is expected.

In my younger days, when I was fit and pain free, I would twist my body by thrashing at the ball. My golf swing consisted of winding the club all the way round my body and then back again. In the process my spine was twisted like a corkscrew as it spun one way and then the other.

Today, I smile when I watch golf tournaments on the television where Tiger Woods performs this same elaborate athletic contortion as he whips the head of his club at the golf ball at an almighty rate. What of course this does to his back is anyone's guess. I have often listened as the TV commentator Peter Allis speak about Tiger after he has once again launched a monster drive up the fairway saying, "Lord, what kind of back will that boy have in years to come?" Of course, we all hope that he stays in one piece for many years ahead. But just what kind of damage is he doing?

As the years went, by I spent more time on the golf course, with the effect that my skills and ability improved. Eventually I considered that I was good enough to play at one of the private courses in the town.

I made application for membership and my name was accepted for the waiting list. Some seven or so years later a letter dropped unexpectedly through my post box. From the secretary of

Kilmarnock Barassie Golf club, the note asked that I make myself available to attend before the committee. On the appointed evening, duly attired in best bib-and-tucker I found myself in the company of other fortunate yet anxious potential golf club members. We were ushered one at a time into the committee room, where a venerable bunch of gentlemen asked all sorts of questions, which scrutinised my right to membership of this prestigious golf club. After some hushed debate among them it was announced that I was fit for membership. I was delighted.

Playing the game to a reasonable standard demands that you must attend regularly. Three rounds of golf per week are expected. In addition one would spend time on the practice ground. But bringing up a young family and starting my own business took away the precious hours that I had set aside for the game that I love to bits. Often after meeting a deadline in the office, I would rush to the course. Having arranged a game with my friends, I would have to change into my golf clothes quickly. In consequence ill prepared, I would then run out to the first tee. After just a hurried few minutes of warm-up, the effort of whacking the ball from the first tee would hurt my cold and ill equipped back. My partner, invariably, would see me clutch at a strained muscle somewhere in my back. But never would I admit that I was in pain. As the round of golf progressed I would aggravate the injury. In consequence the standard of my golf suffered.

At the time, I did not appreciate the damage that I was doing to my body by not warming up. In those days I had no idea of its importance. Now I realise that even when the weather is hot and you feel relaxed you should still warm up for twenty minutes or more before you have any sort of practice swing.

Tiger Woods spends an hour in the gymnasium and then has half an hour of physiotherapy before going anywhere near the practice ground! So, my advice to any would-be golfer is to warm up. You have no idea how important it is.

The warm-up routine that I have written in this chapter is the result of my discussions with a professor of sports science at one of the Scottish universities. I phoned and asked if he could give me some advice on the subject. He responded by telling me that he could. All I had to do was send him £5,000 as the fee for giving me his knowledge. I told him that I didn't have such funds and asked if there was a compromise. Thankfully the professor was a good man and despite the need for the university to show fiscal prudence by earning income from whatever source available to them, he suggested that I should write to him. He asked me to describe in words and pictures the muscles we use when hitting golf balls. Thereafter he would comment on my thoughts. I duly sent in my proposal and waited for a reply. I was pleased when he responded telling me that my warm-up routine was good. In essence I was gently stretching and making supple the majority of the muscles that a person will use when hitting golf balls. I was thankful that the wise professor made no charge for his words of wisdom.

The result is the warm-up routine as written, which addresses most if not all of the muscles that we use on the golf course. Bill Lockie, then the professional at the club, a smashing golfer and now coach to the Scottish Ladies Golf team told me that he was curious as to the format of my warm-up. When I explained the logic behind it he agreed that indeed it did make a lot of sense.

In Scotland we make use of the long summer evenings. Lord knows we don't get all that much good weather, but when we do, we like to make the best of it. Despite the warm weather, many an evening, towards the end of a lovely game of golf, my back would be reminding me that I should have had a proper warm up.

After the game, muscle stiffness would start to set in. Thus I always looked forward to a hot shower. With warm water running down my back it gave me the impression that it was softening the hurt to the muscles.

Sometimes I would stand under the shower-head for ages. In actual fact I was doing nothing to repair the damage. The warm water encouraging the flow of blood to the surface tissue gave me the impression that the muscles as they warmed were relaxing, but this was not so. Much the same as applying a hot water bag to a damaged area it really was a waste of time. As were all of the heated bean bags, poultices, hot rubs and such that my wife would administer when she would see me returned from the golf course, as stiff as an old board!

In this condition I would invariably retire early to bed. But, getting out of bed the morning after a game of golf was an even bigger problem. My back would be rigid and any form of bending would be impossible. In consequence, many a morning I had to rely on my wife to dress me. I could simply not bend down to put on my socks or tie my shoe laces. But life had to go on. Thus, tholing the pain of any movement, and after a little breakfast, I would gingerly get into my car and drive off to work. Arriving at the office, I had to be equally cautious getting out of the car. Not many minutes later I would be seated behind my desk. My stiff back still reminding me how stupid I had been the previous day!

Of course, rather than lying in bed to the last minute, I should have arisen earlier. This would have given me time, to work through some form of early morning warm-up. Then suitably dressed a brisk walk for half an hour or so would additionally soothe my back and further loosen the muscles. Such a work-out would allow the muscle fibres to give, allowing them to relax and stretch, which in turn allowed my skeletal structure to float to where it should be, rather than where it was stuck.

Allowing that 'bones will go where muscles put them', in this relaxed state my structural alignment should be good and in essence I should be pain-free. However, I just never had the time or the common sense for these exercises and so my back suffered.

I have a number of golfing friends. Ex-rugby players among them! Not least of all, six feet six or so of Chris Gray. Chris played rugby for Nottingham and Scotland, and hits the golf ball further than I can. He is a dentist, as are a number of his golfing chums. My delight was to be invited to join them when they set off to play over some of the best courses on offer in Ireland. Some weeks later we flew into Dublin airport. Chris had organised a chauffeur driven bus to take to us to our lodgings in the city. The driver's services would be required over the next days as he carried us to the golf courses we were to play. Imbibing quite a few pints of the famous Irish "black stuff" was our favourite pastime after a game. "Guinness is good for you" - says the advert! With such an alcoholic content in us, none would be able to drive. The chauffeur was an essential.

On the first day of our golf tour we set off for County Louth, a magnificent golf course on the east coast of Ireland. In the weeks leading up to the outing my back had not troubled me. But with pressing work commitments, I had hardly hit a practice ball. I was totally under-prepared. In the locker room I advised that I would have to work though my twenty-minute warm up routine. This was met with derision. A chorus of "Oh what a big Jessie!" and other such words rung in my ears! I was pressed into action without it.

Chris was first to play and crashed a drive, long off the tee. Well to the left, it was more than a bit off line. I hit a more modest shot and dissected the fairway. My neat iron shot to the green was followed by a mercurious putt, and the first hole was won. The second hole and the third I captured also.

The cares of the day and the risk to my back forgotten, I stood on the fourth tee. It was my honour to go first. I thought, "I'll show him". In true Tiger Woods style I launched a ferocious drive up the middle of the fairway.

Much to my shock and to Chris's horror my back muscles went

into spasm. At the end of my golf swing with my club half way round my back, I was stuck. I had torn a ligament, muscle or whatever, causing soft tissue damage. It seemed fairly serious. I stood there more than a little confused. My brain could not understand my trauma. Well, perhaps it could, but it could not communicate the facts with me. Such was the excruciating pain, I collapsed to the ground. Gingerly I rolled onto my tummy. The sensible thing to do would have been to settle in this position for some time and allow my back muscles to come out of the spasm. Then I should have quietly made my way back to the club house. But, what you have to appreciate is that a game of golf is more like a war of attrition. I could not be seen to give in to a little bit of pain. Despite my anguish, I stood up. Gingerly, I picked up my golf bag and walked up the fairway towards my ball. Selecting an iron club I attempted to play a shot to the green. Half way through the swing I dropped the club.

My back muscles were now in deep trauma and my face wrinkled with the pain. I was near to tears, yet my compatriots didn't understand nor did they believe me. It was obvious that they thought that I was using my condition as some sort of excuse not to continue with the game. They were bemused and annoyed that I was now about to upset the format of the golf game for at least that day. I was abandoned where I stood.

When they had gone on their way, I dropped to my knees and crawled to the next tee where I scrambled onto a bench and lay face down. Sweat poured from me. I grimaced with the pain. My brain whirled. I did not know what to do. More to the point I had the shame of not being able to complete the game. I had spoiled it for my friends.

Eventually, along came a kindly golfer. An older chap, he was allowed to take his electric buggy onto the course. I cried out for help. He came over and listened as I explained my situation. He agreed to give me a lift back to the clubhouse. Cautiously I stood on the side of his buggy. As he slowly drove me back across the fairways, I could feel every bump in the grassy surface. It hurt like hell. Worse than any pain I had ever experienced.

An ambulance was called and off I went to the local hospital. On arrival, I remember that I could hardly lift my feet off the ground. The doctor on duty examined my muscle spasm. She gave me an injection into the muscles to calm things and asked me how I had come to find myself in this situation. I explained the golf outing and the fact that I intended to play each day for the next week. Without hesitation, her advice was to get on the next plane home. Indeed she insisted. Unfortunately all of my clothes and my air tickets were in the hotel in Dublin. I was in a bit of a fix. I told the compassionate lady that I would take her advice and would cancel the remainder of the golf. A taxi was arranged that took me back to the clubhouse.

Waiting in the bar at the golf club while the lads finished their game, I tried my best to anaesthetise the pain. I downed copious amounts of Guinness. Later in the evening, in the bar at the hotel, I continued with the same anaesthetising treatment. In the morning my chums had the audacity to ask if I would be joining them for golf that day. I said that I would take it easy for a bit and see if the rest would allow me to play on the next day. (All of this conversation taking place as I lay flat on my back, still in bed). After they left the hotel, I cautiously got out of bed. I could not bend to put any clothes on and had to call the hotel porter for help. The ignominy of having to stand at first naked as he dressed me was hard to take. But the Irish hospitality, his humour, and the fact that he made nothing of my situation, helped.

I was sad that my chums had left me. I was sure that they would be enjoying themselves on yet another glorious Irish golf course, but I accepted that the sensible thing was to cut my losses, get home as soon as possible, and forget about the golf tour. I made a few phone calls and arranged a seat on the next flight to Prestwick in Scotland.

I telephoned my wife to advise that I had cancelled my golf tour and asked if she could collect me from the airport on arrival. From the big sigh at the other end of the telephone I could hear that she was sad that I had wasted my money on something that could have been avoided. Deep down, I could hear her telling me that I should never have agreed to the tour in the first place. I knew that she had resigned herself to the fact that, not for the first time, she would have to care for her invalid husband.

The hotel porter advised that the taxi had arrived at the hotel. He loaded my luggage and then helped me into the back of the cab. In the taxi to Dublin airport, I lay on my back staring at the sky. I was stiff and in pain. The driver was sympathetic to my situation and not at all surprised that my back pain was such that I could not sit upright. He told me that he himself suffered from time-to-time with similar back problems. Then, with typical Irish kindness he suggested that he knew a friendly pharmacist who would dispense some painkillers that might help my situation. There would be no need to visit a doctor for the necessary prescription. Not knowing how I would be able to sit in the plane, I agreed. We set off to somewhere in a Dublin housing estate in search of this pharmacist.

Thinking back, I could have been mugged. I was more than a little apprehensive lying in the back of the taxi when we stopped outside the pharmacy, especially with a gathering of curious children who stared through the taxi windows and looked at me in a puzzled manner.

However, after about ten minutes lying there, the kindly taxi driver returned. In his hand he held two little white pills. He told me to take one immediately, and gave me some water to wash it down with. The other, I was instructed to take just before I got on the plane.

Safely delivered to Dublin airport I made my way to the check-in. There I found a porter who was happy to carry my suitcase and my golf clubs. He made remarks about me having a good trip and such. I was ashamed to tell him my story and yet more ashamed when he refused to take payment for his labours.

The little white pill had worked to the effect that my pain had subsided a little. However, I was afraid that sudden movement would result in a return of the muscle spasm. Soon it was time to board the plane to take me back to Scotland. I was abashed as I painfully, slowly, walked up the steps of the plane. I tottered behind an elderly man who clearly had some kind of affliction. I was mortified to be the mirror image of a man clearly old and in pain. A man with a proper illness! Not the sham of a self inflicted illness that a young man like me should not have.

I suppose one of the worst things about a bad back is that there is nothing visual about it. People are such sceptics about the pretext most used as an excuse for days off work. I had more than a few curious looks from other passengers who did not understand the pained expression on my face. I was in no mood to do any explaining. I only just managed to squirm into my seat, strap on my seat belt, and off we flew. My wife collected me at Prestwick.

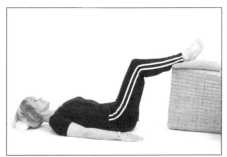 Back in the confines of my own home I adopted a RECOVERY POSITION, lying on the floor (see photo, left), which I found invaluable.

In the recovery position the woman is lying on her back with her hands by her side. She has a small pillow or a rolled-up towel under the back of her head. Having the towel under the head rather than under the nape of the neck allows a free flow of blood to the brain. The feet are placed on a chair or a sofa, with a soft cushion under the heels. In this position the pelvis is tilted slightly backward, which at the same time allows the muscles in the back to relax and rest.

At the time it was the only position that I knew that would offer some comfort. Unfortunately it is easy to get down on the floor but a damn sight harder to get back up. However I have described in Chapter 11 with the help of a couple of photographs a method that I find best.

Indeed a sorry end to what should have been a lovely golf tour; I was quite down-hearted and quite frankly glum. It was quite a few days before I got back to work. I was afraid to venture near the golf course for months. In time my back healed and the memory of my trauma in Ireland faded. Thus it was that the thought of another game of golf was at least somewhere on the horizon.

Scotland is a country blessed with many fine golf courses and I am fortunate to have a collection of business friends who are members of some of them. Invitations to play these good courses have always been forthcoming and despite my troubles I was never one to shirk an offer of a free day's golf no matter how well or badly I was playing. At the same time I had to accept that such an invite allowed that I placed myself into a risk category, with the possible return of my back pain.

Working at the time trying to build my business, I was usually ill prepared for such days of golf. In reality I should have declined these kind offers. My back in those days was never in good condition, but my heart ruled my head and so off I would go.

Stuart Bickerstaff was my most wonderful friend. A kindly man, he was humorous, sensible, a good businessman, a fair golfer, and my confidant in times when a few words of wisdom were required. One day he phoned me with an invitation to play in a foursome at his course. Old Prestwick Golf Club was the home of the very first ever Open Championship and a refined golf course indeed. Stuart was a lucky man to be a member of such a distinguished golf course. Consequently his invitation could not possibly be refused.

He had asked me to partner him in a match against two gentlemen from the U.S.A. Stuart's visitors were friendly business colleagues but his mortal enemies on the green swathes of the golf course. Three holes into the match and "going for the big one," I lost my balance while trying to smash the ball from the tee. Rather than taking a clean golf swing, I smacked the club into the ground an inch or so behind the ball. It did not move an inch. The judder went up my arms and straight to the weak part on my back. My muscles went into painful spasm. I grimaced.

The prudent thing would have been to advise my fellow golfers that I had had an accident. My back was hurt. Sensibly I should have offered my apology and gently made my way back to the clubhouse. But, we were competing in our own mini Ryder Cup! I could not quit. I had a bottle of pain depressants in my pocket that I had taken to carrying with me at all times for just such an emergency. Quickly I swallowed a few, and with, I suppose, a pained expression on my face, continued with the game.

Unusually for Scotland it had been a hot day. My muscles remained reasonably elastic. With more than a little care and the help of the analgesics I was able to manufacture golf swings of sorts and made my way around the course. My contribution to the game was not much. I am sure that on that day I was more of a hindrance than a help for Stuart as we toiled to compete with the visitors from overseas. We did have the advantage that having played such a difficult course so many times, Stuart and I had a good knowledge where to place our golf balls to best advantage. Our American visitors were better golfers but were completely unused to the vagaries and undulations of a truly unique Scottish Golf course. As a result the match finished all square.

By the time we reached the safety of the clubhouse I was beginning to feel pretty stiff. I changed my clothes prior to showering and did so with great difficulty. The fear that one false move would send my muscles into painful spasm made me particularly careful in my movements. Having hurt my back so often, I was now ever alert and prepared for such eventuality. It took time and no amount of engineering to get my socks off. I cannot recall, but would be sure to ask for Stuart's help in the task. Having seen me in such a state many times before, he was not surprised. Gingerly I showered and then dried my aching limbs. With a degree of complicatedness I managed to get fresh socks onto my feet, and scrambled into my trousers. My fresh shirt, tie and jacket made me presentable. Such attire was *de rigueur* for such an aristocratic golf club.

The after match hospitality in the clubhouse was at its usual best. Stuart was a wonderful host. After a jolly good dinner we all enjoyed several alcoholic libations. Enjoyed is perhaps a misappropriation of terms for the alcohol imbibed. Old Prestwick Golf course is exceptional as is Muirfield golf course near Edinburgh which is the home of the Honourable Company of Edinburgh Golfers. Both have the distinction to have the highest usage of a liqueur that would blow your head off.

Stuart had introduced me to the beverage on more than one occasion. However it was akin to drinking rocket fuel. Indeed I remarked on that day as we all downed yet another glassful of the fiery liquid that it had the same kick as the fuel being used by the planes taking off from the adjacent Prestwick airport.

Suitably inebriated we called a cab and set off for home. Sheila was pleased to see me arrive safely but angry that in my happy, intoxicated state I was talking a load of rubbish. I was ushered through to the bedroom where I undressed. More than likely I did not notice that my clothes were strewn in an untidy pile on the floor. I got into bed and soon was fast asleep. Feeling no pain I fell into unconscious slumber. I have no idea for how long I snored. I was oblivious to the fact that she could not get to sleep because of my drunken snoring.

The next day my exceedingly sore head did not mask the fact that during the previous yet enjoyable day, I had indulged more than my fair share of alcoholic beverage. The Scottish saying – 'a heid like a stair heid' was appropriate. I was dehydrated. Indeed my body was crying out for water. With the fascia around my sore muscles shrunk, structurally, I was like a cripple. It took most of the day for my head to recover. It took weeks for my back to recuperate. Ill prepared for golf as I was in those days allowed that my stupidity would result in other days of painful recovery.

I could give many examples of how I hurt my back playing golf. The same reasons seemed to repeat over and over again, yet I was too stupid to realise what was staring me in the face. I was unfit and overweight. I was rarely on the practice ground. Invariably I would arrive late at the course. A proper warm up was out of the question. A few wiggles of the golf club and I would be ready yet physically poorly organised prior to starting a round of golf. These inadequacies were bad, but worse, on the course I would try to make up for my failings by attempting to hit the ball too hard.

In an effort to beat my opponent, or the course, I would attempt to thrash my ball as far up the fairway as was humanly possible. To achieve this I had, as far as I was concerned in those days, to strike the ball as hard as I could. Invariably this would result in a loss of balance. I would have no fluidity in my golf swing. Keeping my head steady was impossible. The result was that often I had the same risk of whacking the ground inches behind the ball.

As with my accident at Prestwick, the sudden jolt with the club head coming to an immediate stop, as it dug into the turf, would go through my whole body. With my spine being at the time twisted and with every bone and muscle in the wrong position, the damage was immediate. Usually the pain was confined to my lower back where five lumbar vertebrae and a big bunch of supporting muscles take the strain, or as in my case they didn't. I knew that playing in such a manner would invariably result in such pain. But in those days I was stupid. Simply stated, I repeated the same senseless acts over and over again. I was my own worst enemy.

Having hurt my back on so many occasions, my fear of pain became an important factor for me to consider. Pain is something that none of us relish and yet it becomes a very prominent issue with back pain sufferers. The thought of the pain when my back muscles went into spasm has often been enough to prevent me from taking the risk of undertaking many a physical act. Playing golf was risky, as were many other manual tasks. I had become more and more afraid that I would hurt my back if I went to a golf course.

Thus after the results of the game at Prestwick, I came to the conclusion that it would be best to stay away from any golf course for a while. In essence I gave up golf and did not hit a golf ball for four years or more.

I retained my membership at my golf club but did not step onto the course. I knew that if I were to relinquish my membership it would take years on the waiting list before I could regain it. I lived in hope that someday my back might just be in a good enough condition to allow me to return to the game that I loved. But I knew not when this would be. I was pretty morose. Perhaps I was a coward.

Eventually as you will see I found the Holy Grail. My life changed irrevocably and my back pain receded. Life returned to normal, or as near to normal as it can be. But the fear factor still lived with me.

I often met Stuart in the pub where we would have a beer and exchange the gossip of the week. He was aware that I had had many months of recuperation. Accordingly he would ask me why, if my back was better, I could not take up the game of golf again. I would always make some weak excuse about being too busy at work or whatever. But it was not the truth; I was simply afraid of my back muscles going into painful spasm again.

But I couldn't tell him. It was difficult to explain such an agonising pain! A pain I would liken at times to having your fingernails pulled out (if you can imagine the pain from such a thing). And so I continued to lie. I was ashamed. I was further humiliated when I could not and did not attend the annual golf outing with all of the lads from the pub where Stuart and I would meet for our regular beer. This situation continued for some years. Then one day I decided that it could go no further. I just had to try to hit a golf ball. If my muscles went into spasm I would just have to admit it and give up the game that I cherished so much. And so one evening as dusk approached, I ventured along to the local golf driving range. At this time of night I knew that there would be few people about. My philosophy was that if I made a fool of my self then there would be no one to tell the tale. I told no one, not even my wife of my intentions.

I warmed up. I spent quite a long time at gentle exercise until I could actually feel the heat from the movements in my back muscles. Gingerly I placed a golf ball in front of me. I held a club for the first time in years. Steadying I swung at the ball. It flew. Not far, yet far enough for me to be content that it had a decent flight from the tee. I had not forgotten how to hit a golf ball, but more to the point my back was not in spasm. I hit another ball and then another. Still my back held up. In all I probably hit 50 or so balls that evening. I stopped and then thought that perhaps a warm down would be a good idea. I went through the same routine as the warm up, packed my clubs and went home. Happy and content I had hope in my heart that perhaps, just perhaps I could return to the golf course. Arriving home I was delighted to let my wife know what I had done. She was pleased. Especially so as the years of inactivity had added more that a few pounds to my weight, which as I have told you is not good for people with back trouble. Getting back to my course for regular games of golf and the consequential exercise could only be good for me.

The next day I phoned a friend I used to play golf with and we agreed to meet at the golf course a few days later. I made sure that I arrived in plenty of time. Parking my car I decided to add to my warm-up routine. I walked away from the clubhouse. I timed that I had walked for ten minutes. I turned and walked back. Twenty minutes in all. It would be my opinion that walking is the best exercise in the world. It uses lots of the muscles, pumps the lymphatics (I will explain later) and gets the cardiovascular system working. It uses just as many calories to walk a mile as it does to run the same distance. (Weight over distance, etc!) When we walk it initially raises the heart rate. This then slows back a little as we continue to walk, but the pressure stays on the heart as the blood pumps. This is good for the heart. In consequence I now agree with all thinking on the.subject that a brisk walk for thirty minutes, five times a week can reduce the risk of heart attack.

Together with a sensible diet it can assist in weight loss and helps encourage a good night's sleep. I find that after a good walk it really does make me feel good.

A stranger to the locker-room at the club house as I was, I was happy that I had gone through my routine by taking the walk. My muscles were warm. I changed into my golfing outfit and began my warm up routine. I was given a funny look by some of the other golfers in the locker room. They were I am sure thinking that I was a nut. Who warms up for golf? Their opinion would be that it was for wimps! However I know that it makes sense and thus I just smiled and offered words suggesting that perhaps for their own benefit, they too should try it.

My partner arrived and readied for the game. We walked to the first tee and set off on our round of golf. I cannot tell how much joy I had playing that game of golf and of course how relieved I was returning pain-free to the clubhouse after the match.

Since then I have probably bored everyone telling them that they should all warm up before they play any game. But I have come to realise that not many people will listen to common sense and so I gave up. Now I just do my own thing. It matters not a jot that I get funny stares. I am happy and content that I am the one with the sense. My golf this year has been good. When I have finished this book I might just have a bit more time to spend on the course and perhaps then I can get my handicap back to where it should be.

I would hope that you will benefit from my experiences. As you can see in my early years I did not know how to live my life. I was lazy. Warm up – Bah! Humbug! Now I know better. It is an old adage, but 'if only I had known then what I know now' then, undoubtedly, I would have been a better golfer than I am today. Certainly I would have saved all of the pain. I hope that you will take my advice.

No matter the sport a warm up before you start is crucial. Many times I have watched golfers at my club who arrive late for a match. They park their cars then sprint to the locker room. Quickly shoving on their golf shoes and grabbing their golf clubs they make their way (much as I used to do) hurriedly to the first tee. They don't have time for a proper warm-up but they make an attempt by having a quick waggle of a golf club. Suitably prepared (or so they think) they then stand on the first tee and whack the ball as hard as possible. In an instant the damage is done and more than likely they will have torn some muscle fibres. Male golfers are too proud to admit that they would ever do anything stupid. Thus despite the fact that they will be in pain we won't hear a word about it.

The tell-tale sign though more often than not will show as the player proceeds up the first fairway. Then you will see him clutching at an area of his back that has obviously been hurt. The damage done on the first tee when cold, tight, sleepy muscles have been instantly stretched by the action of the first golf swing. Mental trauma and physical discomfort! Of course the golfer will pretend that all is well – but the words are not the truth. As their round of golf continues the damage is exacerbated.

Thus I decided that I would fine-tune the warm up routine I designed for the football players to one that would be suitable for golfers. It is this:

In the clubhouse:

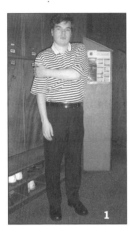

1. Swing the arms across to touch the left shoulder with the right hand.

Touch the right shoulder with the left hand. Repeat each ten times.

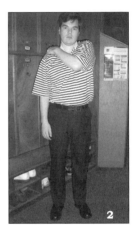

2. Swing the left hand over to touch the right shoulder blade.

Swing the right hand over to touch the left shoulder blade.

Repeat each ten times.

3. Windmills

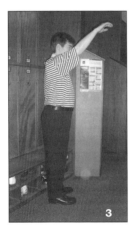

Stand. Look straight ahead. Swing the right arm in large slow circles. Ten forward. Then slow swings in reverse. The inside of the arm should be just brushing your ear as it passes each time.

Repeat with the left arm. Remember a windmill has big slow swings. Don't force or swing quickly! As you swing forward imagine that you are throwing a cricket ball.

In reverse, imagine that you are in the water, swimming the back-stroke. Reach for the water behind you as you swing back.

4. Knee lifts

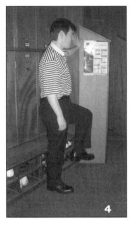

Stand straight. Raise the knee of the left leg without overstretching the muscle. Put the foot back on the floor. Raise the other knee. Then put the foot back to the floor. Repeat ten times on each side.

Each time you raise the knee you should find that the height you can raise would be a little higher, that is until the maximum stretch of the muscles has been achieved. Don't force things.

As with all warm up exercises you should allow the muscles gradually to increase their range of movement.

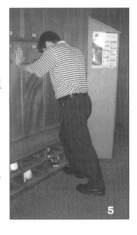

5. Face the wall:

Place the palms of both hands against it and lean in slightly.

Dip to stretch the calf muscle in the left leg.

Straighten.

Stretch the calf muscle in the right leg. Straighten.

Repeat ten times each side.

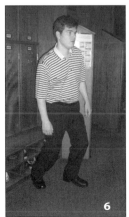

6. Free standing: place one foot in front of the other.

Dip the left knee to stretch the quadriceps. (thigh muscles)

Relax.

Dip the right knee to stretch.

Repeat ten times each side.

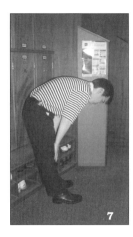

7. Stand straight.

Slowly slide the left hand down the outside of the left leg.

Stand straight. Slowly slide the right hand down the outside of the right leg. Repeat ten times each side. This exercise must be done slowly and gently.

Only allow the hands to travel as far as feels comfortable and pain free, but with each slide, try to slide a little further.

8. Stand straight. Bend the knees a little. Tuck the tail-bone (the coccyx) under, while at the same time gently bending the top half of the body down. Pull the chest in. Drop both hands in front, and gently bend forward running the hands down the front of the legs.

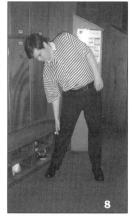

Stand straight. Repeat this ten times.

Each time you bend allow the body simply to fall forward of its own volition. Gradually you should notice that the hands will progress further down.

Continue doing so until the hands can touch the back of the calf muscles on each leg. Exhale each time as you bend forward.

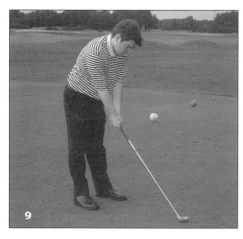

On the tee:

9. Stand holding a golf club with both hands. A driver is best. Hold it out in front of you and place the club head onto the ground.

10. Lift the club and drop it over the left shoulder. Place it back onto the ground in front. Lift and drop it over the right shoulder. Repeat ten times on each side. Each time that you drop the club over a shoulder, raise the elbows and try to touch the back of your leg with the club-head. This exercise encourages the vertebra in the spine to separate, lengthening and loosening the spine in the process.

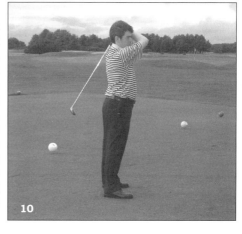

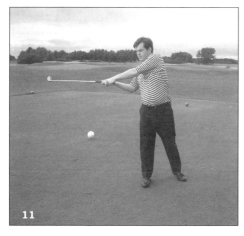

11. Swing the club from one side to the other. Repeat this movement for quite a number of rotations gently swinging form one side to the other, all the time gradually increasing the width of the swing. Continue until there is fluidity in this swinging motion. Continue to swing, but gradually concentrate on increasing the length of the follow through. Of course be careful not to hit anyone as you swing the club.

12. You are now ready to practice a full golf swing, which you should repeat several times.

13. Properly warmed up you are ready begin your round of golf. Line up and keep your eye on the ball and the head steady!

If you love the game of golf as much as I do, you may appreciate that it takes just ten minutes to complete the warm up routine. What you have done though, is loosened the muscles, ligaments and tendons that support the skeletal frame that you are about to twist and turn in a totally un-natural manner. Just like a cat, you should be supple. What you should never forget is that all of our limbs hang from the spine. We control our bodies through spinal movement. As a child we have no control over our spine. We cannot stand. However gradually we learn to control the spine by controlling the muscles around it.

Opening the spaces between the vertebrae in the spine is the key. The joints should not be compacted. Getting the kinks out of the spine will encourage spinal fluid entry. Structurally the two weakest points in the body are the knee and lower (lumbar) spine. The agility of these same points is of the utmost importance to a good golf swing.

What we have done with the warm-up is to energise the body. Energy tells the flesh what to do. Changing the energy changes the flesh. If you are lazy and have a half hearted attempt at the exercise then you will have half hearted energy coursing through your body. Some of the muscles will still be tight. The tension in the body will have an effect on the nerves, pulling and tightening the tissue. You must work the tension out of your body. If you are not in the habit of doing such exercises, in the beginning the movements will be like a rusty hinge. However, in time you should be able to complete the exercises with ease.

Additionally, we have toxins in the body that the blood floods into the brain. When we go through the range of these muscle-stretching exercises we relax the fascia, which in turn loosens the toxins. This must be a slow gradual release. Push too hard and you run the risk of tearing some of the tissue. The soft and supple are disciples of life! The hard and brick are disciples of death!

Research studies of the influence of alternative therapies in golfing are very sparse. What we do know though is that anxiety decreases the ability to focus and cope, which is a requirement for the perfect golf shot. Studies also show that lower back injuries are most common among professional male golfers, while left wrist injuries among professional female golfers.

While golf is not a contact sport, over 50% of touring

professionals stop playing because of injuries.

To consistently play better golf, you must achieve true 'whole body balance'. This means having your body, mind and spirit working together in harmony and balance for every shot. Balance refers to harmony in body organs and systems, in a person's diet, and in relationship with other individuals, society and with the environment. A state of imbalance within one system will affect other systems.

Most athletes recognise that their most important piece of equipment is their body. This entails all the physical characteristics and their state of mind and spirit. The use of alternative therapy (such as I practice) will promote the total well-being that balances body, mind and spirit.

Individuals who are balanced have more stamina and fewer injuries which, if they occur, will heal faster. They are also more able to focus and control the stress response.

Chemical energy results from the food we eat which converts into metabolic energy and provides raw building blocks for repairing and regenerating aging cells in our body. This in turn allows us to be creative, active beings.

We perform best when there is balance and total intercommunication of the different forms of energy. Factors affecting this balance and interconnection are our emotions, perceptions, thoughts, attitudes, ability to give and receive love, and our relationship with God, however we define God.

By the time you have read the whole of this book, I hope that you will understand the words that I am writing, which in turn will make you the better golfer that I wish you to be.

Chapter Ten

WORK

I wonder how some impoverished souls manage to survive a life with back pain, especially so if they have a poorly paid job! Such work will usually involve more that a bit of manual lifting with the risk of back pain that a bank manager or other desk-job person will just never experience. Many men have employment as a manual labourer. Indeed some women work in much the same sphere. Perhaps it may be that they have a repetitive job in a factory processing something mundane. Pressing buttons all day on a machine, in the full knowledge that eventually a robot may well take their job from them. It will replace the need for their manual labour. The unskilled worker has been used and abused for centuries.

I have great sympathy for the impoverished people in the UK. They are at the bottom of the rung in financial terms. Their horizons can only be as far as next week's wages. They cannot afford the cost of private health care. Thus they are at the mercy of the National Health Service. Or, as I have often described it, the 'National Sick Service'! Consequently the mortality rate in such people is high at an early age. Many don't survive the three-score-and-ten that they are entitled to.

These people won't go to the doctor until they are really ill. Eventually when they ask him for help all he will do is offer them a pill to mask the pain. Many doctor's give little, if any, regard to what is actually causing the problem. Thus the patient has no choice but to accept what he is offered. Invariably the patient will have little or no regard for the doctor. For the most part they will just suffer with their back pain. As part of their daily lives they will doubtless be angry that no one will help them. Those in the middle classes may well save a little for a rainy day and will invariably spend what they can afford to investigate their back pain problems. But they also accept that only those at the highest level of earning can have the luxury of a Harley Street doctor, a private hospital or back pain specialist. This lack of understanding of what the patient really needs is surely the reason why we have people off work for long spells. The patients are clients in their doctor's waiting rooms.

But doctors don't seem to see them from that point of view. I am led to believe that the Government in the UK puts restraint on what doctors can or cannot do with their monetary budgets. Telling them when and how they can spend money on the many ills that their patients present. Who knows what sort of regime doctors have to adhere to? But doctors don't share this information with us. Consequently, all but the rich get frustrated. The poor person with real back pain, unable to understand these complexities remains at the bottom of the ladder. Unable to communicate to a grumpy doctor who just won't give the time that it needs to listen, the patient is too often hurried through the clinic by an often more than ill-tempered practitioner.

Too many doctors, it would seem, are irritable. They don't seem to have the time to listen to the patients. Are they just there for the money? I am sure that cannot apply to every doctor, but to me it seems that too many of them simply churn the patients through the system. I hear so many horror stories. Thus I am thankful that my own doctor at least takes the time to listen to what I have to tell. He is a decent fellow.

I have often wondered what happens when a doctor becomes ill. Indeed, are they ever ill? When they are who gives them succour? How patient will they be if one of their colleagues is too crabby to listen to their problems?

I understand that the word 'patient' came from the Middle Ages, a time when there were no doctors. Medicine as we know it today did not exist. Keener on blood letting or covering a body with leeches, the practitioners of the time had much to learn. Our ancestors were the guinea pigs they experimented with. You would be lucky to find someone with skills that could help a symptom. Of course there were some healers who were serious about their task.

They wanted to find ways of making us better. But the only way they eventually found out how to chop off someone's leg without having them bleed to death was to do it again and again. It was only gradually that these early-day surgeons realised that to stop the blood flow from arteries they had just severed required a tourniquet. This learning curve took a long time. Eventually they learned that a tourniquet itself was not good for a limb if left in position for more than a half hour. The control of bleeding was better served by pressing direct pressure over the artery or compressing the edge of the wound. A lot of poor souls were the dummies they practised on. Getting ill had a real risk of death from sometimes the most mundane of symptoms!

In the dark ages if you were a patient, it seemed that you just had to be 'patient' until the pain went away of its own accord. But the basis of what doctors know and understand today was only learned by practising on us mortals. By this somewhat crude method they were able to build a picture of how the human body works. The problem is that doctors spent most of their time working out how all of the main organs in the body perform. Bad backs were a long way from their thoughts. Perhaps though, with the lack of soft furniture combined with hard manual labour in the old days, folk did not have bad backs?

From some of the books that I have read I can see that people who live in places such as Japan don't seem to have back problems. They sit on the floor. They do a bit of manual work every day. They exercise. They don't have soft sofas with piles of cushions on them. They sit on hard furniture. On the other hand, in the west, we have become lazy.

How slothful it would seem that we have become. Most of us don't sit in a chair, we slouch. Allowing our bodies to remain in such a condition for long periods, stores up back pain problems. God just didn't design the human body to be like this.

This slovenly life-style results with far too many people off work with back pain on a regular basis. The cost to Governments around the world is measured in millions of pounds as a cost for people off work with bad backs. Again the rich will have insurance that will allow the best of medical care. They will have probably paid handsomely for it and are able to do so. The poor, on the other hand, have no chance. They are generally too impoverished to afford the cost of the insurance premiums. Relenting to a visit to their doctor they will no doubt be given some medication and sent home with advice telling them to rest on the floor until the pain subsides. Days, weeks perhaps! If they are lucky they might manage to secure a bit of physiotherapy.

But most times, in reality, the folk with back pain who are poor don't have much choice other than to get back to work, bad back and all. They just have to suffer. Filling their stomachs with painkillers leaves them wondering why they have the feeling that the bottom of their stomach is being burned out. Of course it could all be avoided if those in charge of health care recognised the benefits of Bowen Neural Therapy (BNT).

During my working life I have been hurt many times. Often the things that I have experimented with, in an effort to find some solace for my back pain, have hurt me rather than helped. Lots of the systems purporting to be able to help my back pain I found to be a false dawn. I have tried all sorts of so-called cures. The benefit to you the reader is that you might just be able to find the Holy Grail without having to wend your way through the minefield of wizards and quacks that I had to endure. Too many of them were ready and able to take my money while offering me yet another incredible 'cure' for my back problems. Pay some money, take their trick and I would soon be back at work was the offer that I just had to accept.

I am sorry, but the word 'cure' just doesn't exist in my vocabulary. I am at a loss to describe some of the cruel heartless people who offered such succour. Sadly in the days when I was clutching at straws I placed myself in the hands of lots of people who really should be in prison! For obvious reasons I cannot mention who they are. Some of them have made fortunes, yet gave little but false hope to their patients. Hopefully by reading this book you will be able to avoid thcsc pitfalls.

It is a sad reflection on the ability of the National Health Service with regard to back pain, that all too many of us have to scratch about looking for help and relief from our ache. Help it is just not on offer. Thus on my great journey through the back pain of life I have tried most of what is out there. A lot of the time I was searching for the impossible. At times my back pain had me at such low ebb that if someone had suggested that I should drink a pint of vinegar with two worms in it every day, I would have done it. That was until I found BNT, or indeed until it found me. My Guardian Angel guided me towards it. God bless my Guardian Angel!

I have written in more detail about my Holy Grail, Bowen Neural Therapy in a chapter at the end of the book. Suffice to say that it is a system of muscle and connective tissue therapy that helps eliminate myofascial dysfunction. Myofascial dysfunction does not make much sense at the moment, but please bear with me. As I have said I am trying to lead you through my journey in the life of back pain. Stick with me and you will understand why. Please don't rush off to the end of the book just yet. Have the patience to read all of the chapters in their logical sequence. There is a reason for it, as you will see.

Needless to say the cost of a few BNT treatments is minuscule when compared with the cost to the nation in health care looking after people who suffer with back pain. In traditional medicine the treatment for back pain is given after the damage has been done. We don't seem to spend much on preventative medicine, but we should. The Government should. Then we might not have the recourse to call it the National Sick Service.

As you will find I now have a clinic in Glasgow. I am a qualified BNT therapist. How and why I got there will become obvious as you read. But for the time being, be content that I am one. To give an example of what I am trying to say let me tell you a tale.

One day a patient arrived at the clinic with his back muscles in spasm. By profession a scaffolder on a building site: a man who risked his life every day erecting Meccano-like structures around very tall buildings that are under construction. He had as he described terrible back pain. A very general statement! When I asked him to undress I found that he had the worst example of scoliosis I had ever seen. Scoliosis is a lateral curvature of the spine in the thoracic (top of the spine between the shoulders) region. At the beginning of this book I vowed that I would not talk in medical terms, but if you will allow me for this one, I have described on this page the way this man's spine was bent out of shape.

Scoliosis

Lateral deviation of the normal vertical line of the spine which, when measured by X-ray, is greater than ten degrees. Scoliosis consists of a lateral curvature of the spine with rotation of the vertebrae within the curve.

In 80 to 85 percent of people, the cause of scoliosis is unknown; this is called idiopathic scoliosis. Before concluding that a person has idiopathic scoliosis, the doctor looks for other possible causes, such as injury or infection. Causes of curves are classified as either nonstructural or structural.

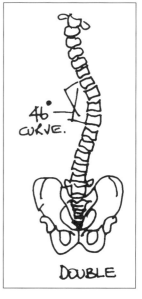

This problem can happen for a variety of reasons. In this man the double curve pattern scoliosis actually helped him to do his work. I was convinced that with his affliction he found it easier to do his job carrying scaffold poles. Long lengths of steel tubes! The tubes were 4 inches (100mm) in diameter and about 12 feet long (4 metres). They were heavy and ungainly. To allow him to carry out his daily tasks the poor man got used to balancing them on his hip. His deformed hip! This was the easiest way to carry them.

What he did not realise was the damage he was doing by putting such strain on the vertebrae (the bones of the spine). Needless to say he ended up one day at my clinic with his terrible back pain. I gave him just two treatments with a week between each. When he came for the second he told me that he was much improved. When I examined his structural alignment I found him to be much straighter. Thus he was pleased to pay for what I administered.

I told him that he would benefit from more treatment but I never saw him again. I had taken the muscle spasm from his equation.

While he probably still had some residual back pain the treatment had taken his pain threshold to a level that was low enough for him to discontinue the treatment and survive without me. A little bit of preventative medicine might have saved him a lot of pain. The man was in his forties, not all that old. His body simply will not be able to take the strain. Gradually he will be able to work less and less. And then he will stop working altogether. What a terrible waste of a skilled worker.

Had we looked after him in his earlier working years he might have been happy to continue working for a lot more years. This would have allowed him to pay his taxes and support his family and continue to be an integral and important part of society. But as the man is today his back pain will progressively become intolerable and thus his working days will be over long before it should be. A little bit of preventative medicine and he could have lasted until his due date for retirement. But because of the Government's stupidity this just won't happen. Preventative medicine just does not exist. As I have said it should though.

If you have a desk job and work in an office, back pain can be just as hazardous. More than likely you will have bad posture. You will be seated with little or no back support. Your knees will probably be at the same height as your hips. You will sit for long periods. If you are a lady you probably sit with legs crossed. You will take a seat in the car or the train or bus on the way to and from the office. Certainly you will have tight hamstrings, (which are bad for backs). You won't exercise. Not even a little. A brief walk at lunch break will probably be out of the question. Especially so if your work has such pressure that requires that you have to work earnestly to keep it. Any sign of slacking and your employer will give you the sack. Thus your nose is always to the grindstone. You will keep at it rather than do the sensible thing and stretch your legs a bit when they need it most. What a disaster!

Most employers are blockheads. They don't have a clue that a little bit of time given to employees each day and spent in gentle exercise would save them a fortune. They are too brainless to realise that if they were to do this that they might just save the cost of staff being off work. Just a little change in work ethics! But employers are greedy. They don't want to see you relaxing, not even for a bit of exercise. Too stupid to realise that in taking all or at least some of the tension and lethargy out of the muscles in your body and that in doing so they will be refreshing your brain. Just a little bit of exercise sets a whole flush of energy coursing through a tired body. The tired brain benefits just as much! Refreshed, you are more able to make sensible decisions. Ones that earn bucks for your employer! If only they would realise it.

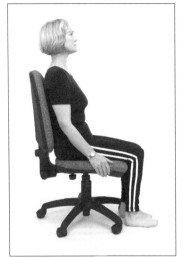

But back to the story! What sensible advice can I give to someone who works in an office? If you have to sit all day then at the very least adopt a proper seating position. Insist that your employer buys you a decent chair, one that will support your lower back! (See photo opposite). Also read the chapter about lifting and sitting.

Perhaps to stay healthy we should adopt the good principles that they have in Japan. Now don't get me wrong: in Japan they have loads of other health problems. Karoshi: death by overwork, for one! But one of the things that they don't seem to suffer from is back pain. What we have to do, of course, is to ask the question as to how they manage this, especially in a country where office and indeed any workers seem to work under such tremendously excessive pressure.

Despite this, as far as I understand it, in some of the offices in Tokyo or indeed any town or city in Japan, on the stroke of every hour a bell rings. Every person in the office, bosses and all stop what they are doing. They stand. Then they go through a short series of gentle stretching and bending exercises. They stimulate the flow of energy around the body.

After a minute or so of this exercise the bell rings again. Then they all get on with what they were doing before the first bell rang. If they were in the middle of a telephone call they simply put the telephone down on the desk and have a pause in the conversation. Of course they can do this because the person at the other end of the telephone accepts that he or she has to do the same thing. Life wherever it is in Japan for that brief moment in time allows that they will all doing the same thing. Exercising!

Even when people in Japan get old this series of exercises continues. All we have to do to confirm this is to have a look at any public park in Japan (or China for that matter). During the daytime they are often filled with old folk where we will find most, if not all of them, going through the routine of the exercises that they learned as children. Usually there is some gentle music to accompany the exercise. Even the children in the schools have to do a set of exercises.

The ritual is hardly pointless. In the offices no one is insulted. They accept it as a perfectly normal part of life. Why we don't adopt this type of goodness in the West is beyond me. The cost saving to the health service would be immense. I have often wondered what the per capita cost of health care is in the UK compared with Japan. I would not be in the least surprised to find that in Japan it is less and more than likely a better health service that we have here in the UK. Why the politicians don't and won't discuss this subject is a puzzle.

And so work has a great bearing on our health. Be it manual or office work we all suffer from the same problems. The type of work that we do just allows that we acquire the problems in different ways. The solutions though are simple. For the office worker we must adopt the Japanese methods. Indeed we should study them. At the very least we should go for a short brisk walk at lunchtime. In doing this we force the healing energy around our bodies. Walking encourages good circulation in a person's body. It will give the heart a bit of exercise. In addition just by walking we pump the lymphatic drainage system. We all have one. It is a system of thin walled vessels found in all parts of the body. These vessels filter off bacteria and other foreign particles preventing bacterial infection from spreading from the tissue spaces into the blood-stream. It keeps us healthy!

If you cannot manage the lunchtime walk then think of something else. If your office is in a tower block then don't take the lift. Walk up a few flights of stairs. Run even. All of this is good for you! (Always check with your doctor before any exercises).

A manual worker probably walks miles very day: climbs scaffolds, pumps the lymphatics, and gives his heart and lungs a good work out in the course of his daily work. But then he spoils it. Never gives a thought to correct lifting procedures and thus hurts his back every time he does it. His employer should be sued. Too many employers never give a thought to explaining to their workers a few simple lessons in the correct procedures for lifting. It should be compulsory. It would save a lot of pain and indeed many days off work.

Thus work takes its toll. Carpenter, plumber, teacher, office worker, nurse or doctor, we all have problems with back pain. Nurses especially have the task of having to lift us in and out of hospital beds when we are ill. Many patients are big lumps of lard. Thus it is no wonder nurses have back problems. We do them no favours.

No matter what style of work we have a lot of us are overweight. Being overweight puts a strain on our backs and more importantly on our hearts. Too much fat around the heart muscle and we are in trouble. But that is another story. In my chapter about good eating later in the book (chapter 20) I have attempted to give some advice on how to lose weight. Not a strict calorie controlled diet. Just a nice way of having a varied menu that may help to keep your weight under control while of course at the same time combined with some exercise.

It is up to you whether or not you take my advice. Some of us have tight work schedules that don't allow us to eat regularly or properly, never mind get energetic. But it isn't as impossible as you might think. A little bit of forethought and you can have the sort of lunch box that your colleagues will envy! Read the chapter.

Work though can be a chore. It was to me. I hated it when I was employed in the construction industry. Some of you out there might like what you do for a living, but I didn't. That is until I first found and then developed my therapy. Now I enjoy my work. I just love helping people to recover from illness and give them some quality in life. However life for me has had more downs than ups! Eventually I came to the conclusion that I wanted to get out of the rat race. I would, I thought be much happier living somewhere like the remote Isle of Barra (an island in the Outer Hebrides to the north west of Scotland). In my dreams, there I would spend my days writing books like this. Or I would spend my time just sitting looking out of the window, dreaming. Perhaps I would spend my time wandering along the white sands on the beach, counting the waves as they came splashed onto the shore. I would be curious to see what interesting items there may be between the flotsam and jetsam, full in the thought that the last bit of land the water touched prior to this was New York in the USA.

In an attempt to fulfil the dream that would give me a chance to get out of the rat-race, I convinced Sheila that we should indeed pay a visit to this faraway part of the world, such that we could experience the life-style at first hand. And so taking the boat from Oban (on the west of Scotland) we set sail for Barra. It was Easter time. The journey from Oban was rough especially when we left the protection of the isles of the Inner Hebrides. The ship rolled and heaved. Many passengers were sick. But the journey was worth the sick bags. The views from the windows high on the top of the ship were fantastic. Scottish scenery is the best in the world!

Arriving at Castlebay, the principal and only town on the island we gazed in awe at the stone church high on the hill above the harbour. Built by the fishermen and women who had populated the island 100 or so years prior, the building of the church was funded by savings from their wages. The wages were hard earned. It was dangerous work as the men set to sea to catch the shoals of herring, which in those days were plentiful. The women toiled for long hours as they first gutted then salted the fish into barrels that were shipped to the markets in Glasgow and London. Sadly the fish are no more. However the church survives as a testament to the backbreaking toil that these people undertook. A big grey stark building, it is built of granite, hewn I suppose from a local quarry. Internally the bare stone walls don't reflect the light. The floor is of hard wood. Barra is a Christian community where church going is very much part of daily life. Thus the building is seldom empty.

Accepting that it was Easter time we agreed that during our visit to the island we would have to see what the church was all about. Before though, we had to carry out some boy-scout work to find how this strange island was composed. We set off in the car. Soon we discovered that there is but one road that goes round the perimeter of this more-or-less circular island. Twelve miles round it didn't take long to go full circle.

We had arranged accommodation in the old school house at the back of the island. Second time round we stopped at our appointed resting place where we would stay for the next week. The next day was Easter Sunday and so after a hearty breakfast we set off for the church in Castlebay.

I was puzzled as we drove round the north side of the island to find a man in a field, digging a grave. I stopped the car and looked. He looked back at me. Not a word passed between us. He was, I suppose, as puzzled as I was at why I would stop to look at him. Instantly he would recognise that I was not a local. He would identify that the car that I had was red and for the time being the only red car on the island. I nodded at him as if to say a silent hello. He nodded back. Scratching my head I got back into the car and we continued the journey to church.

Sunday service was truly a wonderful experience. The women sang the hymns in Gaelic in a soft lilting way that made the hairs stand on the back of my neck. The men, it seemed, were precluded from joining in the singing. The Priest spoke in Gaelic. I could understand just a few of the words he spoke. However as it was Easter Sunday I had half an idea what it was all about. Then the service finished but no one moved from their seats. We decided to sit still. Afraid perhaps to move and make a fuss Shella and I twiddled our thumbs wondering what this was all about.

Then everyone stood. The back door of the church opened. In came six tall men carrying a coffin. At once we realised that we were to experience something unique. Not only were we to have an Easter Sunday Service, but now we were to experience a Gaelic funeral on the same day. Hence the man digging the hole in the ground on the north side of the island!

Needless to say the service was poignant. The hymns were haunting. The eulogy for the woman (as we found out later) who had died was spoken in best Gaelic. I again had not the foggiest idea what the priest spoke about. It was obvious though that this woman had been a much respected pillar of community.

The service ended and most of the folk left with the coffin and headed for the cemetery. The rest of us in true Gaelic tradition set off for the pub. While drinking a toast for the poor woman who had just departed we found that she had been 96 years of age. I thought that she was truly a lucky person. Especially when we discovered that she had been born on Christmas day, died on Good Friday and here she was being buried on Easter Sunday. As a Christian I could see that she had every chance of going straight to Heaven. Her life could not have been better planned.

On other days we explored. We found deserted beaches that had unpolluted white sand. We breathed the pure air. We found and played some golf on the strangest golf course ever. Built on a series of hills to the south of the island the greens were protected by a wire fence that prevented the freely roaming sheep from munching their way through the cut grass on the greens. It was fascinating having to chip over the fence around each green to get the ball near the hole. I smiled as I wondered how Tiger Woods would perform on such a course.

And so for a little while we lived the dream! As part of our week in Utopia, Sheila and I took a flight in a tiny aeroplane from the landing strip on the sandy beach at the rear of the island. This was the fulfilment of a lifetime ambition. It is after all the shortest flight in the British Airways schedule. Taking just 12 minutes from the beach on Barra to the landing strip at the military airfield in South Uist it passed over spectacular scenery.

The captain for our flight that day was a Frenchman. It was amazing when he allowed the plane to tilt to one side or the other such that we could position our cameras to film one beauty spot or another.

A short stop at South Uist for a cup of tea and we were soon back on the plane to Barra. Landing on the seashells on the beach was the most fantastic experience. I would recommend it to anyone.

On the road down to the harbour in Castlebay there was big stone building that had clearly lain empty for years. One night as Sheila and I sat in the bar at the pub, we exchanged conversation and beers with a fellow who was the local plumber. In conversation I enquired as to who owned the building. He pointed me to an old chap with a red weather-beaten face, grey wiry hair and brown tweed jacket who was perched on a stool at the opposite end of the bar.

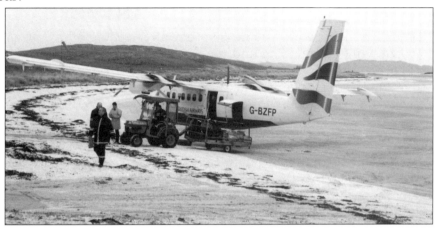

British Airways – Twin Otter. Unloading luggage after landing on the sandy beach at Barra

I had watched as between sips of whisky he puffed happily on his pipe. He looked like a pretty contended man. I wandered towards him not knowing how to open the conversation. I was pleased when he asked me if I was enjoying my holiday. It seemed that he was the sort of man who would know just everything that would be happening on the island. We chatted about ships and the sea. I told him about my father who had been an engineer and who had sailed the world many times. As with many Barra men he had been sea-faring. Thus we had a bit in common. Eventually I turned the conversation to buildings, to property on the island and indeed to the big grey stone building down by the harbour. He told me that he owned it. I asked his price and was pleased to find that the building was available for just a few thousand pounds. I thanked him for the information and told him that I would consider whether or not I could make an offer for the building.

With my construction skills I could see that it could be made wind and water-tight and then completely renovated to our requirements for not a lot of money. I hatched a plan in my head and took the right moment to discuss it with Sheila. My idea was that we would live on the upper floor of the building, while the ground floor would be split for two commercial purposes. On one side I would have a clinic which would open any day as necessary. The other side of the ground floor would be a restaurant that would open Fridays, Saturdays and Sundays. My skills with back pain would be suitable for the one side of the building with my culinary skills being put to use on the other.

Barra was bereft of good restaurants. I am sorry to say this, but sadly it had none. I could see that there was a gap that I could fill. My skills in the clinic would be a useful addition to what the island folk up-to-now had no opportunity to experience. Alternative medicine just wasn't in the equation. The Outer Hebrides Back Pain clinic would be the talk-of-the-town, or so I thought.

Doing my homework I could see that after selling all we owned in Troon, while purchasing and renovating the property in Barra it would leave us with a goodly sum to invest. What I may or may not earn from the restaurant and the clinic would be a bonus. The following day we set off for home. On the boat on the six-hour journey over the fringe of the Atlantic Ocean and back to Oban I could think of nothing other than the idyllic life that lay ahead.

Back home my family thought that I was nuts. I suppose that by then I had cooled to the idea myself and was beginning to agree that perhaps after all things considered it might not just be the grand plan that would make us happy for the rest of our lives. I added up the pros and the cons and found myself in a quandary. I knew that if I pushed for a move to such a remote part of the world that Sheila would eventually agree to come with me.

The remoteness allowed that it would take many hours and two flights to get our daughter up from London to visit. We may not get all that many visitors. On the other hand the island had its own cottage hospital and dentist. The air was clean. The people were nice. The winters would be long, dark, windy and wet but the warm summer months with virtually no nightfall would be heavenly.

Then one day I met a fellow who had lived on the island. He was a patient at my clinic in Glasgow. As I worked helping whatever symptom he had, he told me that despite my good intentions I would end the same as many of the islanders and 'take to the bottle'. In the first months, year even, I would lead a normal life, but in the winter months with short daylight hours I would end up in the pub with many of the other worthies in the island. He told me that the plumber or carpenter or indeed any tradesman were known to turn up for work at 9.00am. They would work until 11.00 and then depart for the pub (for a liquid lunch). Work would re-commence at 1.30 and more than likely be ended at 4.00 when once again they would head for the comfort of the bar stool.

It was suggested that I would finish the same. Having no desire to end as an alcoholic I took the advice to heart and shelved the plan for a life in isolation.

In hindsight perhaps I could have controlled my drinking and enjoyed the Barra style of life. It would have been a laid-back pressure free life. Making decisions on a day-to-day basis without any tension or urgency appealed to me. The decisions of course would be whether to do any work or not. I would be able to take my time. Do what I pleased. Of course in the summer I may have been busy, but I would have six months holiday every year to look forward to. Perhaps the fresh clean air would have been good for my back pain?

But sadly that was not the way that God laid out my life. He has allowed that I have to work to earn a living. It would it seem that there is no easy path laid out for me. Work it seems has been and always will be a part of my daily life. In days gone by work was a chore. Thankfully this is no longer. Now I am happy with life. I am not rich but I have enough to get by with. I have no grand desires. I live a simple life. I have the best job in the world – making people better. Indeed there can be no nicer way to live ones life.

I am a Christian and hope that I am seen as a good one. Aware that there have been some pretty bad ones throughout the ages who professed to be of my faith, I am guarded in what I say about it. Too many people these days it seems are without religion. Cash is their God. Many lead their lives just to make money. The more of it they can make the better. They use and abuse the system, cheat and lie as is necessary to fulfil their desire. Irreligious people! I wonder if they think of what is ahead. Who knows what is out there? What is before us? What happens when we die?

And so as my working days are still with me. But I have come to the conclusion that there is no sense in being a sad sack! My God has decided that I will have to work for a living, so I may as well get on with it bad back and all.

Chapter Eleven

EMERGENCY EXERCISES, CALMING MUSCLE SPASM and OTHER BITS

This chapter is confined to giving a few tips on what to do if you get into trouble.

The worst thing that has happened to me and the most frightening has been muscle spasm, when the muscles in my back contracted and locked up. My system seized. At times the pain was so bad that I could hardly breathe. The first time it happened was on the golf course. I suppose that it was just a twinge, a warning of what was ahead of me. A signal of what was to come in the future. At the time all I knew was that my back was weak and from time to time it ached. Such dull aches and stiffness could last for days. However this new soreness gave me a taste of a sharp piercing pain that certainly made me ask just what was going on inside me.

I have as you know, always enjoyed a game of golf, but as I have explained in my chapter about the game it does put tremendous pressure on my back. Twisting and turning the spinal column like a corkscrew and all in a flash, is hardly what my back was designed for. What damage is it doing? How many arthritic golfers will we see when they get a bit older. Tiger Woods, Colin Montgomerie and other great golfers, as far as I know, have physiotherapy every day. But I would have to ask what is happening to their spines every time they whack a golf ball hundreds of yards up the fairways? Of course these fellows do all of the right things. They are fit and train regularly. They are not over weight. Most importantly they warm up prior to their golf games. And so they have a better chance than the rest of us mortals and are surviving the rigours of their careers without damage to their backs. Or is they? I would like to know. Outwardly they give the impression that they do not have a problem. But I wonder if this is the real story.

I would love to be a fly on the wall in their physiotherapist's room. I wish these chaps the best of health, for all of their lives. But for as long as these fellows are the top golfers in the world, their health will be a big secret to all but their closest aides. Perhaps they have back pain but take daily medication for it. Who knows? It will remain a guarded secret.

Severiano Ballesteros, one of the finest golfers I have ever had the privilege to see in the flesh, has according to press reports, a bad back. In his prime he could hit a golf ball further and with more guile than anyone. In my opinion he was a god. A great champion! A gentleman! A supreme ambassador for the game of golf!

One day, in 1984 I think it was, the Open Championship came to Troon in Scotland. I had a ticket for the second day's play (Friday). I turned up with my sun-tan lotion, and my provisions to see me through the day. Yes, the sun does shine in Scotland! Well at least for a few days in the summer when we probably have the finest conditions in the world for playing golf. Sunny days stretch into the long summer evenings. Playing golf in this type of weather and in the surroundings that we have the luxury to enjoy can be described as nothing other than – gorgeous! It makes me dribble to think about it. Better than sex. But back to the plot:

I had enjoyed a good day. I had positioned myself at a variety of advantage points around the course. I had relished watching the good and the great. Wondrous golf shots all day. I was sun tanned and happy. I had been able to luxuriate in something special being so close to all of these stars. The day was drawing to a close and thus I was starting to think of making my way home.

I headed for the seventeenth tee. As I walked up a grassy slope towards the teeing ground that was slightly elevated I could hear the noise of a party of golfers approaching from behind and could hear the stewards asking the crowd to stand aside to allow the golfers through.

What happened next will live with me forever. The great man brushed past me. His arm touched mine. My hair stood on end. I was shocked and stunned. I stumbled after him trying to gain a vantage point, to watch him tee-ing off at this par three hole. He took a few practice swings. Then with the greatest of ease that only the finest of golfers can manage, his ball flew towards the target. Of course his shot was superb. It landed softly. Plumb in the middle of the green, just six feet from the flag. I was in awe. Dumbstruck!

Sevvy (as he is known fondly) and his caddie walked away from those of us gathered around the tee and set off across the lush fairway, which had been so lovingly prepared by the green staff at this illustrious golf club. I followed as best as I could pushing and shoving through the throng that was by now attempting to get a view of what was about to happen on the green. I cannot remember if he sunk the putt for a birdie as I could not see past the crowd that had thronged around the green. I wasn't disappointed though. All that mattered was that he had touched me. I was sanctified.

As you know I am married to the blessed Sheila. A good woman, she has looked after me throughout our marriage; I owe her much. In reality after such a glorious day on the golf course I should have made my way home to tell the tale. I love Sheila and the two lovely children we are blessed with. But, being the man that I am, probably the man that most of us are I decided that rather than being a sensible person and returning to my family, I should go to the pub and relate the tale to the boys at the bar.

A few beers later and my mates were fed up with my story. I had vowed never to wash my arm, well at least not for many days. I was touched, or so I thought. Perhaps I had just had too much sun!

I have followed Sevvy's career through the good times, and the bad. He has been a revelation. At the Ryder Cup, a few years ago, the bi-annual battle between American and European golfers he was an immense player. As captain of his illustrious bunch gathered from most of the golf playing countries in Europe he was a true leader, in every sense. Despite my absolute admiration for the man, it has always grieved me that his back has troubled him over the years.

I have heard a tale that one time when he was over golfing in Scotland his back was sore. In pain he was just like the rest of us. He looked for something that could offer some relief. Anything that would make his back just that little bit more mobile and able to hit the golf balls he had to. Of course he urgently required something to stop the back muscles going into painful spasm. I heard that he was advised to visit a chap in a wee village not far from me. The man (some sort of bone cruncher) performed his tricks on his back, but from what I heard I don't think that it worked. Sevvy was at the time just like any typical back pain sufferer willing to clutch at straws no matter how little the chance of success. Like many of us he never questioned the man's credibility or his qualifications. The therapy he administered wasn't proved or evidence based. But more of this later!

At times when I have been in pain, I suppose that if someone told me to stand with my feet in a bucket of horse manure with wet fish sticking out of my ear, I would probably have done it in the hope that it would give me some succour from my back pain.

Despite his problems Sevvy has managed to carry on golfing.

Today he is not the golfer he used to be. Father time catches up with everyone. He still has his back pain. When he was in his prime I wish that I had been able to speak with him, just to share the muscle calming exercises that I will now share with you.

In the days when I was an old misery guts I was unaware of the myriad forms of alternative medicine that are available around the world. However one day a man who was aware of my back pain told me about a book. It was entitled Treat Your Own Back and was written by a fellow called Robin McKenzie, physiotherapist born in 1931 in Wellington, New Zealand. I managed to find a copy and read it from cover to cover.

I consumed its contents in just a couple of evenings of speed reading hoping to find the panacea my back ached for. I then experimented with the exercises he described. However I came to the conclusion that I could not agree with much of the book no matter the excellent credentials the gentleman appears to have. Indeed I found that some of the exercises he explained hurt me more than helped me.

I was about to give up when I turned to the back of the book to what he called the 'panic page'. There I recognised an exercise that my old yoga teacher had taught me years before. It did seem to make sense, especially so when McKenzie seemed to agree. And so every time my back muscles went into spasm I got down onto the floor and completed the exercises. It was for a long time my only support. With it I managed to take the spasm out of my back muscles. A bit of 'do it yourself' physiotherapy it is described in the next set of exercises.

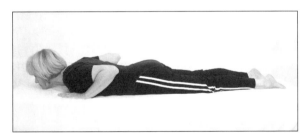

Photo (a): Lie on the tummy. Place the hands as shown to either side. Look slightly ahead.

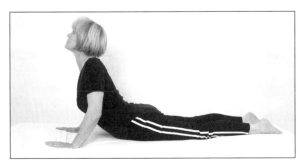

Photo (b): Push to straighten the elbows, at the same time keeping the hips firmly fixed on the floor. As you raise the torso from the floor, exhale while raising the head to look just above the horizontal. Only raise the back as far as is comfortable and pain-free. Hold for a few seconds and then gently return to the floor. Rest for a few seconds with the head turned to one side taking slow deep breaths. Repeat the lifts and rests a number of times.

McKenzie developed his own method for the treatment of back pain and spinal disorders. He has had some of his writings published in the New Zealand Medical Journal and has published four books on a variety of medical subjects. While he has to be congratulated for what he has written and undoubtedly what he has done for many back pain sufferers around the world, his form of treatment does not seem to get to grip with the problem. His treatments are as far as I am concerned a 'slow boat' method of recovery.

In my opinion if the problem were chronic, the patient would not be able to perform half of the things that he suggests in the book. At the least, most of us would be afraid to attempt them for fear of making things worse. Thus while I found his book to be of value, it was not my holy grail.

I don't think that I need to tell this to a back pain sufferer, but in conjunction with the exercises as explained it does make sense to take things easy for a day or two. Later in this book I have written a chapter about how to get in or out of bed, how to carry and lift things, etc. It is important that any back sufferer accepts that he or she will have to change things in their life. Get out of all of the bad habits. Once you have experienced the Holy Grail (HG) you will manage to do most of the things you could as a child. Your mobility will return.

It is really worth understanding the myriad of things that are out there suggesting help for back pain sufferers. The Internet, for example has a load of junk about 'cures' for back pain. My advice would be to leave it well alone, until at least you have read this entire book and had a chance to experience some BNT. With the knowledge that I hope you will gain from this book you will then have the wisdom to laugh at the stupid things that people sell to the unsuspecting public. Pills, rubs, corsets, chair supports and other such implements don't, in my opinion, have one bit of value.

'Cure' of course is a word that I will never use. People who come to my clinic get help. Pretty damn good help, but that is as much as I want to describe it. The vast majority of my patients are happy that with BNT I can take them to a good level of health. Some of them are hardly 50% when they come to me. I may never make them 100%, but they are happy at 95%, especially if they can avoid surgery.

The emergency exercises and muscle calming is thus as I have described. I cannot find a better form of it in any of the multitude of textbooks out there. McKenzie is correct and rightly so has reproduced it in his book. But perhaps we should be having a closer look at what Yoga could do for us. I accept that there are many Yoga exercises that could do more harm than good; however I find that by sifting through things at times you can come across a gem, much as McKenzie has offered.

When attempting the exercises it is difficult for any back pain sufferer to get down flat on the floor to do the work. More to the point how to get back onto your feet when you have completed them can be troublesome. So, let us role-play. Pretend that I have just wrecked my back by stupidly lifting a bag of cement. My back muscles have gone into spasm. I am wracked with pain, sweating, with my mind in a blur. Unable to think straight! Worse, let us say that there is no one in earshot to help me. What will I do?

As I have said the first time that it happened to me was on a golf course. Probably it was a moderate form of muscle spasm, if there is such a thing and thus I was able to walk from the golf course, albeit with difficulty. I got some one else to carry my clubs. Gingerly, I managed to get into my car and drove home. When I got there I was able to hang onto things in my living room as best as I could and use them as crutches such that I could get onto the floor. I set myself in my recovery position as shown in chapter 9.

In this position my back is flat on the floor and is where in this position in time my muscles will calm. I suppose it did help to take some painkillers. The problem as I found is that the overuse of painkillers eventually seemed to burn a hole in my stomach. It is disturbing to read a recent report as written by the Spanish Centre for Pharmacoepidemiological Studies in Madrid. They used the UK General Practice Research data base to compare the risks for those taking NSAIDs with those who were not.

Typical of these types of drugs are ibuprofen, naproxen, diclofenac, indomethacin and meloxicam. Heart failure, a relatively common condition in the elderly, arises when the heart no longer has the ability to pump blood effectively. The Madrid team reported that that taking NSAIDs increases the risk of getting heart failure by 30 per cent, after other factors are taken into account.

Of the NSAIDs, indomethacin seems to carry the greatest risk, tripling the chance of hospital admission with heart failure. The study did not look at the modern alternative to NSAIDs, called COX-2 inhibitors. Vioxx, one of this class has already been withdrawn for increasing the risk of heart attack and stroke in a trial. Many patients with osteoarthritis need NSAIDs to make life endurable, so the extra risk of heart failure is unlikely to change their habits. But the study does emphasise the need for powerful painkillers with fewer side-effects.

It didn't take a University study to convince me that taking handfuls of pain-killers wasn't a good idea. The pain in my tummy told me enough to know that I was doing no good. Now that I have my therapy I don't need any pain relief for my back pain. Indeed I even have a simple BNT remedy for the odd time that I have a self induced headache.

Leaving the painkillers aside I would recommend that if you have a back problem and cannot get some immediate therapy to help then it is good to spend some time first in the recovery position and then gently turn over into the abridged cobra position (lay face down and rest on your elbows). The cobra is useful when reading or watching television, however I find that it becomes tiring after a while. But alternating from the recovery position to the cobra can be a reasonably comfortable way of spending an evening when recovering from a back muscle spasm.

Last, but not least, when I went through the years before BNT I found that it was possible to get onto the floor when I hurt my back. The ever more difficult bit was getting back up. I had to lie there for long periods as it was the only route at the time to recovery but sometimes I was in such pain and so unable to move that I found it impossible to raise myself from the floor, even to get to the toilet. Many times I had the ignominy of having to ask my wife to get me a bottle to pee into rather than go through the trauma that would be involved in trying to stand straight. I accepted that I had to get onto my feet again but had to do so in a way that wouldn't hurt. As you can imagine I attempted all sorts of contortions to get me back onto my feet. With the benefit of my experience I would suggest the following instructions to help.

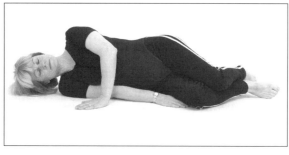

I would normally find myself lying on the floor but adjacent to a sofa:

(a) If you are lying on your back pull the knees up and use the quadriceps (the big strong muscles on the front of the leg that join the hip to the knee) to push you onto your side such that you are facing the sofa.

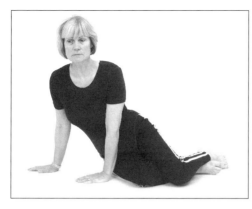

(b) Push up to the side using the arms as levers

(c) Gradually pull and push to get into an erect position kneeling position. Then begin to push with the muscles in the legs, while holding on to the sofa, using it as a prop. Gradually rise from the floor until you are in a standing position. It is of extreme importance as you rise from the floor that you keep looking up. I cannot understate the importance of looking up when involved any activity involving getting to an erect position. Stand for a few minutes taking a few deep breaths before moving off.

Protecting your back of course is tantamount to survival, so you have to think about it all of the time. I find that getting in and out of the car can be fraught with danger, and so I developed a simple technique. Getting in, first open the car door as wide as it will go. Hold onto the roof of the vehicle and slowly lower your bottom onto the seat. At this point you will be facing outwards. Settle into the seat. Keep your knees together and slowly swing them into the car. Pull the door shut. Put the seat belt on. Getting out is the reverse: this time when raising yourself from the car seat, use the strength in the legs to do the lifting. At the same time hold onto the car and push yourself up with the arms. You should be able to manage it with a bit of practice.

I find that it is best when driving a car to keep the legs bent and the back supported. This puts much less strain on the back. It is of course essential that when driving that you don't stay in the same position for long periods. If I have a long journey I will stop at least once every hour. Get out of the car and do some exercises and then walk up and down a bit, before continuing the journey. This gets the circulation going, and keeps the energy flowing around the body. I would also suggest that you carry out a series of 'knee lifts' and 'windmills'. (See over) This simple set of exercises will stimulate the sleepy blood that has been stagnating in the lower limbs by encouraging it to circulate around the body and become re-oxygenated. Thus it will travel to all parts full of healthy nutrients. In addition to refreshing the muscles it will awaken the brain and pump the lymphatics.

Knee lifts

Hold onto something (a door handle or whatever) to steady

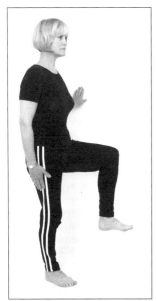

yourself. Gently raise the left knee as far as it will rise comfortably. Lower to the ground. Repeat on the right knee and then the left again. Continue with repetitions on each side, alternating. As you do so, feel the muscles in the thigh (quadriceps) stretch just that little further, allowing the knee to rise a bit higher each time, until that is that you have achieved the maximum stretch of muscle.

Windmills

Swing the arms in big circles, ten times in a forward motion, and ten in reverse. As you swing, allow the arm

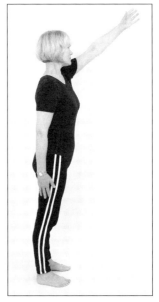

to brush past the ear. In the forward swings pretend that you are throwing a cricket ball. In the reverse swings, imagine that you are flat on your back in the water and are swimming the back-stroke, each time reaching for the water behind you. Remember that the swings must be slow. There are quite a number of shoulder muscles to be moved. Windmills in Holland go slow, so, please don't swing fast, like a propeller. The muscles just don't like it and won't respond the gentle stretching that you are trying to encourage.

I don't find that there has been much good reading or informative information in most of the books written about back pain. Many books are written in language that most ordinary people cannot understand. In addition, I often wonder if the person writing the book had a bad back. Having never suffered back pain, I don't see how you can understand how debilitating it can be. This is probably why I decided to write this book. Just by putting things in a little better perspective and in words that the layperson can understand, I hope that it all makes sense. As far as muscle calming and emergency exercises are concerned I hope that all that I have written will be of help. Indeed I hope that you agree with me that all that I have explained makes sense and will be of comfort to your back as you make your way through life.

Chapter Twelve

BAD BACKS,
THE VIEW OF THE GENERAL PRACTITIONER

I had always wondered what is in the mind of a doctor when someone like me makes an appointment and, arriving at the surgery, blurts out the age old platitude, "I've hurt my back." Will the doctor be able to differentiate between the person with genuine back trouble and the likely lad, who has convinced himself that the doctor will not be able to detect the ruse he is trying to play, just to secure a few days off work? Well, to get some answers, I approached my own GP and put some questions to him. I was surprised at the answers.

The unwritten doctor's bible, in the first paragraph says, 'eyes and mouth first, hands least and last!' What does this mean? Well more or less as it reads. 'Look and listen'. My doctor always comes into the waiting room to invite his patient into his room for a consultation. Why does he do this?

The answer is, to see how the patient gets to his feet from a sitting position and to see how able he or she is to walk to his room. By simply using his eyes, he can tell a lot from this. Did the patient take his time to stand? When he stood up, did he do it gingerly? When he walks, does he do it briskly, or can he hardly lift his feet off the floor? There is a medical term for "dropped foot." It is too big a condition to include in this story, but what it means is that there are nerves from the back, which join to the feet. These nerves basically make you curl your toes. If the nerves in the back are hurting, then you cannot do this, and so in a way you are tripping over your own feet. All of these little pointers tell the doctor about the patient, before he has even opened his mouth.

There then follows a series of questions and answers. In this the doctor is trying to work out the history of the problem. How long have you had the pain? Where exactly is it? What is it like? Is it worse when you do this or that? Every doctor has this stock list of questions to ask, before he comes to any kind of conclusion.

Doctors are taught at medical college to build up a mental picture when someone presents a complaint. In building up a picture of the problem, they are looking for associated components. Are there any aggravating factors? Does the back get worse when you bend? Is it worse when you walk, or is it worse when you lay flat on your back in bed? Can you lift things? Can you put your own socks on? Can you get behind the wheel of the car and lift your legs to change gears? Relieving factors are also important. Does it get better when you walk or sit, or indeed is it better when you lay on your back on the floor? Are there any other times when it gets better, or is the pain constant all of the time? The answers to all of these questions allow the doctor to build up a mental picture of the patient's complaint. Observation is the name of the game. Look at the movement.

I spoke of a slipped disc earlier (and the fact that the disc doesn't slip); if the patient is able to walk normally then "it is not a slipped disk." A disc is anchored in place, but most people are familiar with this term as the main cause of lower back pain, when in fact this is only true in less than ten percent of back troubles. You can imagine a disc as being roughly circular in shape and having a tough outer shell and a soft gel like centre (a fibrogelatinous pulp - see sketch). This, like all other parts of our body needs nourishment, but if our back is rigid through lack of exercise, then the flow of nutrients into the disc will be slow. To improve this, it is necessary to have regular exercise. This is why it is important to take a brisk walk every day, and of course make sure to wear well-cushioned footwear when you do it.

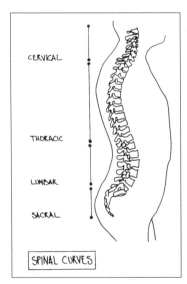

SPINAL CURVES

After examining movement a doctor will then have a look at the curvature of the spine. It should have a natural "S" shape to it. A lordosis: the natural inward curvature in the cervical and lumbar regions of the spine. (see sketch). There can be a number of reasons that cause malfunction, with ankylosing spondylitis being a culprit. However I find that when the spine has straightened and there is nothing more sinister causing it then more than likely the back muscles will be in spasm. When this happens, I reckon that he will be able to tell just by the pained expression that you will have on your face. That has certainly been the case with me, when I have had a muscle spasm. The pain when this happened was such, that it made me weep is something that you will not want to happen often, indeed, not at all if you can help it.

There are other circumstances, which can give you back pain, but they are not related to the muscle or bone type of pain that we are trying to discuss in this little book. In any case the chances of you having them are slight and they would frighten you if I told you about them anyway, so are best left alone. If you are in any doubt, ask your doctor. As I have been trying to explain here, he knows a lot more than you give him credit for.

Of course doctors do get people at the surgery who are "at it", but there are other factors which can exacerbate the problem. For example, if a patient is depressed, then he will likely have a lower pain threshold. One would think that loading the body axially would be a sure sign that the spine and the back are under pressure when in fact this is not the case.

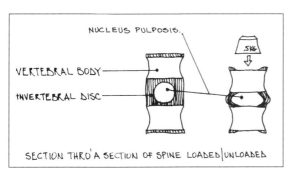

SECTION THRU'A SECTION OF SPINE LOADED/UNLOADED

Rotation or the lack of it is a more salient point. The spine is made up of two main portions, the upper section, which is fairly rigid, no matter which way you move or bend, and the lower portion, which does all of the rotation. This is why most back pain is in the lower back.

To catch out the likely lad, the doctor may ask the patient to lie flat on his back, with the legs straight in front. He would then try some straight leg rising. No doubt the likely lad would complain that it hurts when he does this. The give-away, is when it comes to sitting up. If you are really in pain, this will be difficult to do. Sitting up straight is not a good thing for the back if it is hurt. It is also near nigh impossible to do if your muscles are in spasm. The likely lad however in all probability will be able to sit up quite easily and gives away the fact there is nothing wrong with his back. If on the other hand the patient is rigid on the couch and has no curvature on the spine, then there is not much doubt about it.

It is a sad fact that old age is something that comes to us all and this is when we suffer from wear and tear, some more than others. Post-menopausal women can suffer from collapsed vertebrae, but not all of them, mind you. Your doctor will be able to give explicit advice on this subject and I am sure some medication to cope with it.

As I am neither female nor post-menopausal, I will miss out on this one. If you are a lady reader, and you have this condition, well I am sorry for you. If you are a man, well it's time you were washing the dishes and doing some of the chores for the good lady!

Painkillers! Yes we are all sceptics when we are offered them to dull the pain. How many times did I come away from the doctor thinking that he gave me painkillers just because he could not be bothered to examine me properly and this was an easy way for him to get rid of me? How wrong I was and how little did I know or understand. Drugs make you tired and slow you down and if you are tired you will rest. Rest calms the muscles, which may be in spasm; more painkillers make you tired again and so on. In other words a virtuous circle! Less = less.

Acute pain used to be treated by traction in hospital, but this does not happen so much these days. This form of treatment involves you lying flat on a bed. Weights hang from a pulley with a series of wires, which are attached to the ends of your legs. The gentle pull from the dangling weights pulls on the ends of the legs. In essence, a stretching of the spine! Reminds me of what they used to do in the torture chamber in the medieval times.

The sacrum is the big bit of bone at the bottom of the spine; it has flat plates on it, which join to the pelvis. The pelvis is the big bit of bone, which forms your hips. If you overload the ligaments in this position, the muscles become inflamed and then the doctor will give you some anti-inflammatory pills to dampen down the heat in the joints, as well as the painkillers. If there is a lot of spasm in the muscles, the doctor may well give you an inoculation, or a small dose of muscle relaxant pills to be taken perhaps for a day or two.

Surgery depends on the nature of the problem. It has to be a joint decision between the doctor and the patient. The patient and the surgeon would decide on a management plan, but sometimes it can make the matters worse. If for example you have a 50-50 chance of success, is it worth taking the risk?

Modern surgical advances now have a system called chymopapain chemo nucleolysis. Sorry to use big words again, when I had promised not to, but basically what the surgeon will do is to inject the middle of the disk with a liquid much like pineapple juice, the enzymes of which dissolve the soft gel centre and thus the prolapse of the disc (the bit bulging out), is helped.

This may well save the need for a laminectomy, a type of operation to be avoided. This involves opening the back to remove the bits of bone, which can be pressing on the nerve at the back of the spine. It doesn't sound like much fun to me. So, here's a cheer to the good old pineapple juice. (Funny, but I have always used pineapple to tenderise gammon steaks in the kitchen).

The surgical procedure in laminectomy is complex. We have five discs at the bottom of the spine. The middle two are fused and the spine then becomes rigid. This happens as the 100% movement that you used to have in five discs, now has to be achieved in the three discs left. What an engineer would call, a biomechanical problem. Taking bits of bone from the hip and packing them between the discs achieves the fusion. The bone chips work like an adhesive and gradually fuse the two discs into one rigid piece. In all something that I would submit to as an absolute last resort!

The words in this chapter give view of back problems from the GP's point of view. Not what I thought it would be. If anything, it has shown that they have a difficult task, when confronted with someone like me.

Doctors are not stupid, and while you may think they are not giving you the best of treatment, in fact your health and a cure to your ill, is their only aim. The fact is though that they don't have x-ray eyes.

Nevertheless, I hope that these words throw some light on their workings. It certainly confirms in me that doctors are all natural optimists, and worth their weight in gold!

Chapter Thirteen

AND HERE'S WHAT TO DO IN BED!

How often do we consider the merits of the piece of furniture that we spend a third of our lives tucked up in? Some pretty important events take place in the thing. Fun, conception, birth, illness, death! You can add to the list yourself.

The house in Ardrossan where I lived as a lad had three rooms (living-room, bedroom, front parlour) and a kitchen. It was on the ground floor of a tenement – a block of flats. The Scottish word 'tenement' describes a sandstone building that contained flats (houses). Two on the ground floor, two on the first floor and two on the second floor! In all, six families survived in cramped conditions. There was one toilet on each floor, located in the close (corridor) between each house that we had to share with our neighbours.

Our kitchen sink was pressed into use for all sorts. Pots and pans were washed during the day! Legs, arms, feet, face and hair at other times! The mother of the family that lived next door used to carry out her ablutions standing in her sink. It was a regular event on a Friday evening. As a young gullible lad it put a smile on my face as I would sit on the garden wall with my chum and view her exertions. It was a real eye-opener! The plastic window curtain did little to hide her vanity.

The living-room in our flat had a coal fire. It had a back boiler that heated the water for the kitchen sink. The fire was great to sit around on a cold winter's evening. However it wasn't much fun when it was my turn in the cold frosty mornings to go and chop kindling, carry in pails of coal and set the fire, while the rest of the family were still warm in bed.

Despite the difficult living conditions, it was a happy house and a nice place in which to live.

My parents slumbered in a built-in bed. A Scottish invention, the bed was located in a cupboard just off the living-room. To most folk in those days it would be known as a 'concealed bed'. During the day the door of the cupboard would be kept closed. Those who came to visit were left un-aware that my parents slept in this cubby-hole.

The living-room was the centre of all family life during the day. A place where every bit of family life was acted out and of course the room where I grew through the early years of my life.

Early one Christmas morning I crept through to the living- room to see if Santa had managed to leave me some presents. I think that I was about five years of age. You can imagine my puzzlement to find my father sitting up in bed. In his hands he held the book that I expected to find in my stocking, filled with the goodies from Santa Claus. Why he was reading the book that was to be part of my fun later in the day I never fully understood. I don't think that he ever properly explained why he came to be holding it. "Taking a wee loan of it" – I think were the words he used to explain.

Apart from the living-room that housed the cupboard and in it the built-in bed that my parents used, we had a small bedroom that I shared with by brother. My sisters slept in another built-in bed in the parlour (the front room). The parlour was the pre-eminent room in the house and kept as a reception room for visiting family and friends.

In those days we didn't have television. People made their own entertainment. My parents had many friends who often came to visit on a Saturday evening. They brought their children with them and bags filled with bottles of beer and whisky for the men and port wine for the women. They also brought along a variety of musical instruments. The children (and me) would hide behind the sofa in this big room where we would intently listen to the adult stories.

Sometimes we would wrinkle our brows, unable to understand the words our parents would use. We were though happy to be regaled with these stories especially when there was so much laughter.

The songs and music from a variety of instruments that the visitors would bring were a joy to listen to. My Uncle John Tinney was a wonderful singer and a marvellous exponent of the mouth-organ. He had them in all sorts of sizes. From a tiny instrument that he could hold between his teeth and play by pursing his tongue and blowing through what seemed to be impossibly small orifices in the instrument, to a giant of a mouth organ that was more like a mini keyboard. This monster seemed to take hours to slide from one side to the other. No matter what he played the sound was for ever magnificent. He was a very gifted and skilled man. I am sure that he could have given Larry Adler a run for his money.

These were happy times. The adults were content with their friends. The beers and whiskys would be followed with big platefuls of mouth-watering sandwiches. The children would snaffle a few of the sandwiches and some of the cakes and biscuits that accompanied them and have our own picnic behind the big sofa. We were lucky to have such a life style.

At the end of the evening the children would be packed off to sleep in the built-in bed in the parlour. Sometimes there would be six of us in the bed. Boys and girls mixed together, we slept top to toe. Three heads on pillows at either end of the bed. What fun!

The bed itself was similar to most if not all available in those days. An assortment of springs hung between some steel rails that rested on wooden slats screwed to the wall. On top of this was a horse-hair mattress. It was comfortable as far as I can remember.

However, frugal Scots were known to be sleeping in this sort of arrangement long after bed design and manufacture had moved ahead considerably. The resulting holes, lumps and bumps in mattresses would not do much for any of us suffering with back pain. Yet some silly Scots would rather suffer than put their hand in a pocket to buy a new bed. Even today I can think of many a Scot's farmer with short arms and deep pockets who would rather suffer with back pain, than spend a few pounds on a decent sleeping solution.

Beds of course have been around in various forms for many years. Bed covers have evolved with them. I once visited the Weston St. Francis hotel in San Francisco, California. Apparently it was the first hotel in the USA to have sheets on the beds. (Prior to this the guest would use the horse blanket that they would bring with them). In many countries and for many centuries the bed was considered the most important piece of furniture in the house. In ancient Egypt beds were used not just to sleep in but also to eat and to entertain socially.

The earliest beds were shallow chests into which some bedding was placed. The mattress was a bag of soft filling more commonly straw but sometimes wool. In the 18th century the cover was made of cotton and by now the filling included coconut fibre, cotton or horse hair. It is said that the Egyptian pharaoh Tutankhamen slept on a bed made of ebony and gold, with a comfortable mattress filled with goose feathers, yet his subjects would sleep on palm boughs heaped in the corner of their home. Despite all the wealth in the world today I wonder how many poor unfortunates still have to sleep on such an arrangement.

By the time of the Renaissance the more affluent would have mattresses made of coarse ticks, which were stuffed with feathers and then covered with sumptuous velvets, brocades and silks.

My visit to the Palace of Versailles (to the south of Paris) confirmed that Louis XIV was fond of the ostentatious and ultra spacious variety, wherefrom he would hold court. The beds that I viewed at the Palace were enormous. There must have been lots of kitchen-maids scurrying about their Lords and Masters' bed chambers on a cold winter's evening, rushing to place the polished copper bed pans that contained hot cinders under the crisp sheets.

The expression 'sleep tight' of course comes from the 16th and 17th centuries when mattresses were placed on top of ropes that needed regular tightening. In the late 19th century latex mattresses and pocket spring mattresses were introduced. The first coil spring for bedding was patented in 1865.

As a boy I can remember the iron bedstead being part of the flitting (the furniture removal) when people moved house. Every family had these sorts of beds. The polished timber bed ends and the rails that joined them together were one thing that they would take with them. The coiled spring could be replaced when worn, but the 'bed-ends' often manufactured from hand carved and highly polished wood would go from house to house. In time the bed-ends would be handed down to the next generation. Today the same bed-ends can be found in some of the nicest houses, although the coil spring and straw mattresses that hung between are now being replaced with modern high quality mattresses.

Today technology allows us to have a choice of inner spring mattresses, upholstered foundations, futons, foam rubber mattresses, modern water beds and air chamber mattresses. Memory foam is the latest technological advance, not to mention the high-tech adjustable sleep sets that can manoeuvre the occupant in all sorts of positions. People taken to hospital with serious burns find it painful when lying in bed in the one position.

The air chamber mattresses for such use are manufactured from memory foam, but with a succession of holes drilled through at regular intervals. This allows a steady but gentle stream of air (with the oxygen it contains) to be blown though the holes and onto the patient resting on it, which in turns helps the healing process. The mattress is the most important part of your bed. Good advice is to spend as much as you can afford. When you spend more, you'll gain deeper filling, which will provide more comfort and prolonged mattress life. Most mattresses contain some type of spring system deep inside and generally speaking the more springs a mattress contains the greater support it will offer. Whilst sprung mattresses are by far more common, there are now other types such as, slab or solid latex, or memory foam (visco elastic) mattresses which offer an excellent alternative. Some beds have a combination of good quality springs and a layer of memory foam. Perhaps the best of both worlds!

My wife and I decided to purchase a new bed earlier this year. Allowing that I practice-what-I-preach, I could not allow the current version to outlast the ten years that it had resided in our bedroom. My wife in any case was starting to complain about a 'funny noise' that it made when she was going to bed each evening. The springs on her side of the bed seemingly haven given out, and thus it was indeed time to dispatch the bed (that had been to now a good servant) to the bedroom in the sky.

However before embarking on the parting with some of my hard earned currency, I decided to do some research. I was more than pleased to be offered the opportunity to visit the Sealy factory at Aspatria in Cumbria, a charming little town in the north of England, some twenty miles west of Carlisle. I had visited it some years ago when I was the President of Kilmarnock Rugby Football Club. We had taken a team down for our annual 'friendly' match. Not that any rugby match can be described as friendly. "Honest, I didn't mean to burst your nose, but let me buy you a beer" would often be the topic in the bar after such a match.

My recollections of the visit were a bit hazy due to the fact that when we arrived at the Aspatria rugby ground, their President was delighted to tell me that for the duration of our stay, the drinks were free! Aspatria (God bless them) were a team of hardy lads; farmers and such. In that season they had made their way through the various rounds of the Pilkington (a big serious glass making company) Cup, to the extent that they managed to survive to the quarter-final. For a junior side, this as a massive achievement! There they played the mighty Wasps (from London) Rugby Club.

The match had been held the previous Saturday. Needless to say just about the whole of Cumbria had turned up for the most important match for many a year. The game added a lot to the history of this little but so socially and generically important rugby club. Aspatria did their best but lost narrowly. The benefit to the club was the income from the massive crowd who came to view this wondrous spectacle.

The takings at the gate and of course at the bar and the numerous temporary bars that they had opened at the ground for the day had resulted in a wondrous inflow of much-needed cash for this little club. The fact that they had made so much money meant that they were flush (well at least for a few weeks!!!).

And so Kilmarnock RFC turned up the next Saturday.

Unknowingly, we were to be the recipients of this generous Cumbrian hospitality. They wanted us to share in their good fortune. Something that I have come to know and cherish with folks from these parts! I don't know whether we won or lost. The hospitality was such that I slept all the way home to Ayrshire.

Quite a few of the lads who played for the team worked in the 'bed factory', they told us in the after-match banter. I had no knowledge that such a thing existed. Out here in this beautiful countryside was the last place that I would expect to find such an industrial unit. Yet here it was! Down the road to the back of the rugby club, tucked away in a valley was this massive factory where lots of the local people worked. Rugby players! Wife's of rugby players! All sorts of happy people!

With thirty years of successful business behind them I suppose that no one understands beds like Sealy. Based in this lovely part of Cumbria but with the back-up of the world's most advanced testing laboratories in the USA it is a grand place in which to work. As you can imagine, it produces a first-rate-product.

The Sealy technicians work with leading orthopaedic surgeons to develop the Sealy unique, advanced sleep system. The latest technology and nature's most luxurious materials provide unsurpassed comfort and support. Sealy bed customers, include prestigious hotel chains, high profile celebrities, the wee man from Ayrshire writing this book, sports stars and even royalty across the world, who all appreciate waking up feeling refreshed and full-of-life.

A bed can be a costly item. In reality it should be the most expensive piece of furniture in a house. Yet how many of us give it the importance it deserves? We spend so much time in it, yet give little consideration to this fact. With my bad back I spent hours in the thing that displayed itself as my resting place many a day. I tossed and turned. Talked to God! Asked him why he had afflicted me so. Cursed! Ruminated! Squirmed with pain! Wondered why it was me who should have been inflicted in such a way.

When my back was bad, how many hours I spent in bed is beyond recognition. I didn't count. Of necessity I was just glad to get my aching back onto something comfortable. I didn't give a thought to the lumpy and oft-times bumpy camp-bed-of-a-thing I spent all these hours in. Too many times I crawled into the object with no thought of how long I would be there. In those days my brain was quite simply out-of-gear. Unable to think straight I often just lay there exhausted. My back pain was all encompassing. The bed had just always to be there. It was my crutch. I hated sleeping on the floor. I was ever angrier at the advice from the doctor who told me that sleeping as such would help me. Today I question his wisdom.

But when you are young, in your teenage years you don't get lessons on where to purchase a bed. Your mum does that sort of thing, doesn't she?

Then you get married. Have a lot of fun making a family. But totally oblivious to the fact that the bed that Auntie Jessie (or whoever) bought you for a wedding present was a well-meant but cheap-as-chips bequest that in fact was doing more harm than good.

Despite this you sleep in the damn thing for more hours and days than is good for you.

I don't know of anyone who has written about sleeping positions when you are in bed. However with the knowledge that I have garnered over the years I will offer some advice. The first and most important words are the ones that repeat every day in my clinic. "Look up and Stand up". To explain:

When folk get up in the morning, no matter the condition of their back they will swing the body to the edge of the bed and struggle to an upright position. Now perched on the edge of the bed, normally with elbows on their knees they will rub their eyes, stare at the floor and ruminate as to where their knickers (underpants) are. Eventually coming to the decision that they will have to stand they will begin in this bent position and will push forward. Gradually, unthinking, sometimes abruptly they will ascend to a standing position. In the process the centre of gravity will be way ahead of the body. The consequential strain on the back enormous! The words 'ouch!' will often be heard. The 'sore back' has just reminded its inhabitant that it is still there. Waiting to pounce at the least sign of stupidity!

The correct way to get in and out of bed is explained in the following chapter. A good piece of advice, it will take you safely through the years. After a bit of practice, much like all of the healthy and prudent exercises that I have described it will change your life for the better. Once learned you will never forget. Please take this advice and have it be with you as an integral part of life, for whatever years God decides to give you.

When my back was painful and long before I found the therapy that I now practice, I developed a sleeping position that seemed to help sooth my aching muscles when I was trying to sleep. Sudden movement in bed when your back muscles are near to or just recovering from spasm is risky! Getting into and out of bed (as shown in the next chapter) had its own risks. Nevertheless, taking my own advice when arising in the morning I would sit at the side of the bed. Then I would look up. Just above the horizontal is sufficient. In this position I would then use the quadriceps (big muscles on the thighs) to help me arise. But, whoa! I can hear you ask. Why look up? What is this all about?

Without writing in anatomical terms let us accept that the spinal cord contains all of the nerves that are dedicated to sensory and motor control of the limbs. An adult spinal cord is 45 cm (18 inches) in length. It has a maximum width of 14mm (0.55inches). The spinal cord continues to enlarge and elongate until an individual is 4 years old. Up to that time enlargement of the cord keeps pace with the growth of the vertebral column. After the age of 4 the vertebral column continues to elongate, but the spinal cord does not. Suffice to say that I find the subject of the spinal cord, the arachnoid mater, the dura mater and indeed the sectional anatomy of the spinal cord altogether fascinating and altogether to do with the therapy that I now practice. However the subject is complex. Suffice to say that the spinal cord is contained in the spinal column and in a way moves along inside it.

The point that I am trying to make is that it is like a bit of elastic inside a tube. If you bend the tube the elastic has to stretch. In a stretched position the already inflamed and agitated spinal nerves can become even more so. By bending your head forward as you look at the floor when you arise from bed, you in fact bend the tube and stretch the nerves in it. By bending forward (as most people do) as we attempt to stand first thing in the morning, the spinal nerves are stretched ever further.

Alternatively with the head in an elevated position (looking slightly above the horizontal) the nerves are not stretched, but relaxed and then less likely to complain. The sketches in the next paragraph explain this in more detail. I hope that it makes sense. It will certainly make a difference to you if you suffer at all with back pain. As you grow older and become infirm this bit of advice will stay with you and be of help.

Of course once in bed it is important to lie in a comfortable position, especially if you are going through a period of back pain. From the drawings in the next chapter you will see that when we get into bed at first we are on the side.

Gently one should turn onto the back. Then making a decision about which side would be more comfortable to lie on I would then turn carefully to the selected side. In this position I will then pull my knees towards my chest. In this way I will be in the fetal position. Much like a baby in the womb!

Fetal development starts at the ninth week and continues until birth. The skeletal and muscle systems are formed in the first four months of gestation. Safely tucked up in a mother's womb a baby will be most times happy, content and pain free. In the fetal position most joints are flexed.

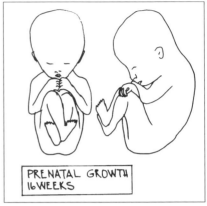

In times of back pain, I like to return to this happy and comfortable position where my aches and pains can fade away as my body rebuilds itself and the

Sketch of a baby in the fetal position: prenatal growth at 16 weeks old.

muscle and soft tissue regenerates. I find also that if I read in bed that it is better to lie on your side with the book propped on the pillow beside you. Lying on your back with the head twisted forward to stare at the pages of a book I find does not do one any favours.

Lying on the left side may be more beneficial that lying on the right when sleeping. I have no medical proof. However my reasoning is that the blood in the heart flows from the right atrium and ventricle and is pumped into the left atrium and ventricle before it pumps the blood back into the systemic system.

It may be nonsense but I consider that it is slightly easier for the heart to pump the blood from right to left (top to bottom) as you lay on your left side. Lying on your right side, in theory you are asking the heart to pump the blood up-hill.

Unlike most other muscles, the heart never rests. This extraordinary organ beats approximately 100,000 times per day, pumping roughly 8000 litres of blood-enough to fill forty 55-gallon drums. Despite its impressive workload, the heart is a small organ, roughly the size of a clenched fist. Thus it is my intention to do everything that I can to help it. I accept that during the night everyone twists and turns as they sleep. However whenever I get the chance in the few minutes that I am awake I will always return to sleeping on the left. The breathing exercise (again in the next chapter) will also help to take the pressure off the heart. Give it a wee holiday. As with our whole body we only get one heart so the more that we can do to help it, the better.

Of course before you arise from bed, before you are weight-bearing it can make good sense to carry out a series of back exercises. Please again refer to the next chapter for this advice. I find that in bed first thing in the morning, in a relaxed state, the muscles are happy to co-operate and stretch when you ask them to. By the way in the morning when we stand up you will find that we are all an inch or so taller than we were when we went to bed the previous night. During the night at sleep in bed, the discs between the vertebrae have time to relax and become spongier and fluid filled. The gap between the vertebrae widens a little. Adding all of these microscopic changes together allows that we find ourselves this inch (25 mm) taller. Of course during the day as we go through our daily duties gravity is pulling us towards the ground, with the result that the discs get compressed, loose their fluidity and microscopically shrink. Thus when we get to the time to go back to bed in the evening if we were to measure our height we would find that we had shrunk by the same inch or so.

The better the bed of course, the better the sleep! Sleep is important in that your entire body relaxes, and activity at the cerebral cortex is at the minimum. Heart rate, blood pressure, respiratory rate, and energy utilisation decline by up to 30% allowing the body to regenerate and rebuild and for our energy levels to recover. Shakespeare described sleep as 'the chief nourisher in life's feast' although research has not yet identified specifically what sleep does. Napoleon, Florence Nightingale, Margaret Thatcher and others survived on just four hours per night. There is of course no set amount of time that a person or an animal requires. I am happy with six hours per night. A sheep on the other hand requires just 3.8 hours while a python will sleep for 18 hours each day. Perhaps it can be best described by saying that the amount of sleep that we require is what we need not to be sleepy in the daytime.

If we don't get good night's sleep we seriously affect the brains ability to function properly. With sleep deprivation the part of the brain that controls language, memory, planning and sense of time can virtually shut down. This can have a major impact on congenitive functioning and also on our emotional and physical health. Sleep and sleeping disorders is a subject of many other books. Suffice to say that good advice is to give your body the best chance that you can to allow it to recover, which in turn takes us back to the quality of the bed that we sleep in.

I don't use my bed for mental activities as I accept that need to associate my bed with sleep. I go to bed at a fairly regular time such that my body clock is synchronised with my desire to nod off. I would never watch television in bed although I have done sometimes when I have been away from home at a conference or such like. In such a situation when I have been away from home on my own I would get bored. But I found that watching the TV made me tired in the morning. Apart from that, what I watched as with most TV was a load of rubbish. Now I take a good book with me. Go to bed at my usual time, read for a wee while and then I'm off to sleep. When in a hotel I usually find the rooms stuffy and most times would turn the heating off.

I find that this helps me to sleep. Hotel beds can be good and other times downright awful. Thus I am always glad to get back to my own bed.

The bed that we have just renewed was ten years old. I accepted the aches and pains in the morning were partly due to the age of the thing. Replacing it was a sensible move as after ten years the resilience can deteriorate considerably. Having absorbed sweat and skin over the years the dust mites in my bed would be thriving on a feast. An asthma sufferer would never leave a bed such a long time as the debris from one's own body can create a breathing hazard.

The last bed we had was a 4 foot 6 inch wide bed. In reality it gave my wife and I as much room as a baby's cot. The new king-size gives us more space to sleep together. We are happier in our own space. There are many types and prices of beds to choose from these days, each offering its own features and benefits. However my advice would be to spend as much as you can afford. It's probably one of the most important investments that you will make, not just for your home, but for your own well-being. In reality every £100 that you spend represents just 10p a night over 10 years.

The three main elements in a bed are springs, upholstery and filling. There are many ways in which these can be combined making price and choice very wide indeed. Factors such as your weight and build will determine the level of support that you need. It would be my opinion that a bed should be neither too hard nor too soft. Supportive enough to keep your spine straight but soft enough to cushion your body too!

Thankfully in later life, I appreciate the necessity, indeed importance of a good bed. Especially so, if like me you suffer at all from any form of back pain!

I hope that you will take the hint.

Some useful web addresses that may help you select the bed that will be most suitable for you:

www.sealy.co.uk   www.bettersleep.org

www.sleepcouncil.com   www.allergyuk.org

www.backcare.org.uk   www.britishsnoring.co.uk

Chapter Fourteen

SURGERY and DISC REMOVAL

In the time of my deepest depression, when I had come to the conclusion that the doctor was correct and that a life in a wheel chair was all that was before me, I had time to think. Believe me at night I did a lot of thinking. When one is suffering from such debilitating back pain, there is a lot of time to ponder. At night in bed when I was tossing and turning, trying to get some sleep, my back pain ruled. Just as I found a comfortable position and I was relaxed I would begin to drift off into deep sleep. The muscles, which had been fighting my every move all day, began to relax. The stiffness started to go out of my body. My sub-conscious would begin to take over. Calm descending I was travelling into the land of dreams. Then all hell would break out. Relaxed as I was my sub-conscious mind would decide that the restful position I was in was not good enough. Thus in my sleep my body would move. Not in the protected way that you have been doing all day, but in an involuntary way that used the bits of my body I had been trying to preserve when I was awake.

And so in an instant I would be awakened with that oh so familiar pain. The top half and the bottom half of my body were trying to turn as I slept. Unfortunately they forgot to take the hinge in the middle with them. The tender, sensitive, unprotected portion of my lower back!

And so my back muscles would be once again in spasm.

The pain would hit me like a bolt of lightening. Instantly I would be awake. My restful sleep gone! Not that I had had much of it in any case. Sometimes I would hardly have been asleep for fifteen minutes or more. However in my perilous state at that time fifteen minutes was indeed a long time. Thus in the middle of the night I would be awake. I would settle back to the comfortable position I had left my body in before I had drifted off to sleep. This time though I would be afraid to go back to sleep. And so I would lie awake and think.

My brain would churn and I would first think of the words that the doctor had told me. From then and for the rest of my life I would have two choices – live with the pain and the muscle spasm that invariably would come more often and settle for life in the wheelchair. Alternatively submit to the surgeon's knife. Wondering what the surgeon would do was bad enough. The wheelchair was perhaps a better option? Immobile, dependent on others, my life would have to change. How would my friends view my circumstance? Would they be forgiving? Would they help me cross the road, indeed would they open the door to the pub? How would I drive my car? Who would dress me in the mornings? What happens when I go to the toilet? Who wipes my bum?

Oh Lord this is not good. Too many questions! How am I going to be able to cope? Worse! Will my wife desert me? I will become a burden. Sex with the woman I love will become difficult, indeed will she want to make love to a cripple? Oh help, my life is tumbling down around me. Suddenly life in a wheelchair does not seem so attractive after all. What am I going to do? And so you think a bit more.

Surgery, is this the answer? No matter how awful it may be, it might just have to be. And so you ruminate. What are the risks? Is it painful? Will I still be able to walk after it? What if the surgeon's knife slips when I am on his table? Suppose he is more interested in the new blonde nurse in the operating theatre and what he is planning for her after work, rather than the important matter of sorting my back. Oh blimey this is not good. What am I going to do?

And so night after night, for weeks, I went through the same format of gingerly going to bed, drifting off to sleep and then abruptly wakening. Each night, the same thoughts raced through my head. I was going mad. It had to stop. I had to do something about it. Thus I began some research.

I am no expert in back surgery. My knowledge is exceedingly limited. However I set myself the task of finding out. I began to ask questions of each and every doctor and nurse I could lay my hands on. Sadly the conclusion seemed to be the same. They all gave me the same answer. The success rates in back pain operations are not good. Indeed the rates are bad. Only a 25% of people have a chance of complete recovery. Some poor souls are left paralysed. This did not auger well. But then I thought of the alternative. The wheelchair!

Oh crivens, what was I going to do! I could not allow things to drift as they were doing. Each day my back got worse. I got myself into more and more tight spots where I had to cry out for help. I was fed up having to ask my wife to dress me in the mornings. I was ashamed that I had to ask her. Worse my work was suffering. I was becoming less able to complete my daily tasks. Soon I might have to pack in my job. No longer would I be the breadwinner. My family would have to survive on much less income. No more nice food. Neither holidays abroad nor trips to the theatre! Dinner out in a restaurant would become a thing of the past. This is awful. What am I going to do?

Suicide?

Yes of course I considered it. I thought about it on more than one occasion. Very carefully turning matters over in my mind it was a real option. However the coward that I am when it comes to things like this precluded me from taking it to the wire. On the rugby field faced with a brute that was just about to kick me in the head or the bollocks or indeed anywhere where it would hurt I would do my damnedest to defend myself. In a dark alley on the way home from the pub with three thugs intent on stealing my wallet I was the bravest fighter you could ever imagine. But taking one's own life, gosh that was a different kettle-of-fish.

After a time I accepted that suicide was indeed the coward's way out. It would destroy my family. What would they think of me? They would never forgive me. Apart from anything else, as a Christian I would go to Hell. No, sorry it was out of the question. I had to find something else. And so in my waking hours I decided that I would have to do yet more research. Just how bad was the risk in back surgery? What could I do to cut the risk?

In my research I found Hugh Owen Thomas (1874). The father of English speaking orthopaedics, he suggested that rest was the cure for back pain. Long periods of it were best. He came from a long line of Welsh bone setters. Thomas incorporated many of the bone setter's manipulative skills into the orthopaedics treatment of fractures and dislocations. The discovery of the ruptured disc in 1934 allowed orthopaedics to dominate back problems. (Orthopaedics – The branch of surgery concerned with disorders of the spine and joints and the repair of deformities of these parts). Surgical fusion came later.

When the Second World War came along, it gave orthopaedics even more scope for experimentation. Combined with improved health care, generally, orthopaedics became the leading specialists in spinal disorders. Or so they said. Sadly 'Joe Public', you and me, just had to go along with their findings. We had no choice. Well we did, we could go back to Thomas and accept his advice for bed rest. In the 1950's there was an explosion of disc surgery, which was closely related to neuro-surgery. However this was not without its problems. In America the situation was made worse by the question of liability. Who was to blame if the surgery, as it often did went wrong? Who did the patient sue? The medical fraternity then came to the conclusion that spinal fusion might be a better answer.

However despite the fact that surgeons now have all sorts of high-tech equipment to help them with the task, the simple back pain problem is still with us.

Could it be that too many of us submit to the surgeon's knife when an alternative, simpler, solution may have sufficed? We are able to complete all sorts of spare part surgery these days. In time most bits of our bodies will be 'off the shelf'. The back though remains a complex problem and for the conceivable future would seem to have to stay that way. In this modern world that we now live in, we all look for a 'quick fix' when it comes to medical problems. Sadly when it comes to back pain back there is no easy solution.

In all of this we have the 'fear factor'. Afraid of what will happen to us if we don't have the surgery and at the same time afraid of what will happen if we submit to it. Fear is a basic instinct throughout the animal kingdom. Afraid of walking home in the dark, fear of the big dog at the end of the lane and so on are all the same family.

Why are we afraid? The answer of course is that we are afraid of pain. We all have an extreme loathing and dislike of pain. However it is a very natural happening. Submitting to the surgeon's knife might be painful. What would happen if the anaesthetic didn't work and we woke up on the operating table? Blimey would that be painful! Fear though has a useful purpose. The best example that I could give would be a child touching something hot. The sudden pain instinctively has the child withdraw the hand, thus minimising the damage. Sadly it is not possible to do this with back pain. It creeps up on you. You have an impending feeling of doom. You can feel that it is about to strike and there is sod all that you can do about it. You just have to accept and get on with it. Suffer!

And so it takes us back to my conflict of wheelchair or surgery. The inordinate amounts of time that I lay awake at night thinking about it, going over the same topics again and again went on for months on end. The worse the state of my back on any particular day, the more I would think about it at night. The more I would have restless sleepless nights.

All through this period of my life I spent my time visiting one quack after another. On each and every occasion I had the hope, and the wish that they would resolve my problem. Give me a life without pain. Sadly, as you will have realised from various parts of this book, which relate to these trips, I got no respite.

If I did, it was always a short term fix. Thus surgery and disc removal in my opinion were out of the question. Unless you have something really badly wrong with your back it has to be the last resort and would be so only after exhaustive discussion with your doctor and surgeon. Indeed was I to consider such a drastic step, I would be inclined to discuss the subject with more than one specialist. The wheelchair with all its associated problems would in my opinion be the better alternative. Although neither is really acceptable! That was of course until I found the 'Holy Grail'.

Chapter Fifteeen

MUSCLE SPASM

This is a difficult chapter to write in a manner that makes sense. How the body works is a science all of its own. However I consider that it is important for the reader to have half an idea how the body works in relation to muscle spasm and back pain. Physiology as I have discovered is a fascinating subject. I can see that in essence we don't know half of what goes on inside a human being. When we eat food we put into our mouths and then just forget about. What the body then does with it and indeed what comes out the other end after it has been though our own chemical factory I find amazing. Yet the more answers I get about how things work inside us the more questions it poses. However in as simple words as possible let me explain a few things that I consider that are relevant to a human being suffering with back pain and aching muscles.

The human body contains trillions of single cells. Every day millions die and are replaced by millions of new cells. To work efficiently these cells must co-ordinate their activities. The combination of different cell types creates tissues – collections of specialised cells and cell products that perform a relatively limited number of functions. There are four basic types of tissue:

Epithelial tissue that covers every exposed surface of the body and forms the surface of the skin, lines the digestive, respiratory, and urinary tracts. In fact they line all passageways that communicate with the outside world.

Connective tissue fills internal spaces. It provides structural support for other tissues, transports materials within the body, and stores energy reserves.

Muscle tissue, which is specialised for contraction. It includes the skeletal muscles of the body, the muscles of the heart, and the muscular walls of hollow organs.

Cartilage and bone are called supporting connective tissues because they provide a strong framework that supports the rest of the body. The body contains three major types of cartilage with fibrocartilage being particularly important. It is located in the pads within knee joints; between pubic bones of the pelvis and intervertebral discs. Its functions are to resist compression and to prevent bone to bone contact. Injuries to these joints can produce tearing in the fibrocartilage pads that does not heal. Eventually, joint mobility is severely reduced. Surgery generally produces only a temporary or incomplete repair.

Neural tissue carries information from one part of the body to the other in the form of electrical impulses.

Telling a little about tissue may help you understand a little about the body. However, as I stated at the beginning of this book I don't intend to make it into something that you won't be able to comprehend. Skeletal muscle is important to people who suffer with back pain. It is the voluntary contractile tissue that moves the skeleton. It is composed of muscle cells (fibres), layers of connective tissue (fascia), and numerous nerves and blood cells.

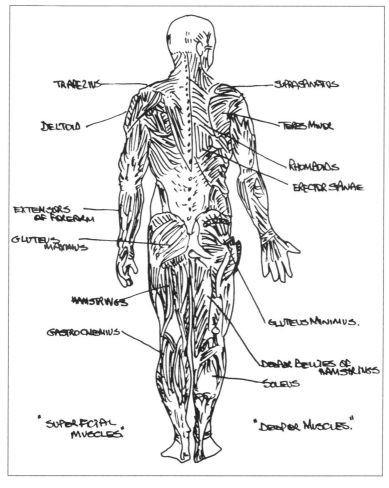

Sketch of a skeleton with an explanation of most of the more important muscles

Muscle is the most abundant tissue in the body and accounts for some two fifths of the body weight. We cannot exist without muscles. Indeed it is impossible to do anything without them. The chemical components of muscle are intricate, and too complex for this book. Suffice to say that when we decide to do something, make a movement, whatever, the brain works out what we want to do and sends a signal normally to groups of muscles at the same time. A chemical reaction takes place and the muscles shorten.

Muscle tissue is unique because it can be in a relaxed or contracted state. When a muscle is relaxed it has a soft, malleable feel. When contracted, it has a firm, solid quality. As the tension in muscle tissue changes, surrounding tissues like tendons and fascia also become taut or loose.

Who you are and what you are is expressed in muscle language. You can use the muscles in your mouth and tongue to speak, or you can use the muscles in your arms, hands and fingers to write words. You can dance. You can run or swim. You can use your muscle to fight your enemy.

Muscles are the engines that your body uses to propel itself along. They don't work like your car engine, but they do the same sort of work. Your car needs petrol to make it work. It converts it into energy. The food we eat, the protein, is turned into fuel for our muscles – 'energy'. The muscles turn this energy into motion. Muscles are vital. Muscles are clever. They are able to repair their own tissue. They last the length of your life. If you are an athlete the muscles can be trained to grow strong. They do everything from allowing us to walk, to keeping our blood flowing.

Muscles use energy in the form of adenosine triphosphate (ATP). To make ATP, the muscle does a variety of wonderful things that convert the oxygen we breathe in and combine it with the glucose, fats and amino acids that we eat into ATP, water and carbon dioxide that we exhale. I had occasion last year to be asked to speak at a fund raising luncheon for a local charitable organisation. The dinner was attended by about 250 women who were mostly past the prime of life. I did my best to explain the strange yet wonderful therapy that I practice and answered as many questions as possible in the half-hour that I was allowed to speak.

Finally a wee woman stood up and asked me if I could do anything for energy. She told me that she had none. I told her about ATP and how she, indeed all of us, makes it every day. I also told her that when she stopped making it that they would put her in a box with a lid and not let her out for the week-end. I don't think that she was too impressed nor did she have half an idea about ATP despite the fact that it is crucial to our survival.

After death, calcium levels inside the muscles grow and the bodies level of ATP drops. Then the wonderful things that our muscles have been able to do for us throughout our lives stops and the muscles remain in a contracted or stiff condition. This state is called rigor mortis. When you are dead of course you don't need your muscles and indeed for once your back pain will be gone! However for the moment let us concentrate on the fact that we actually do need our muscles.

Muscles and fascia determine the body's shape. Facia is an important part of the body. Like tendons and ligaments it is the fibrous dense connective tissue network located between the skin and the underlying structure of muscle and bone. It keeps everything separate within us. To explain it simply I would ask you to think of an orange. Peel the skin and you are left with segments of juicy flesh. Each segment is wrapped in a thin layer of membrane. This is much like the layers of fascia, which separate all of the bits of us inside our bodies.

We have fascia just under the skin: a superficial layer attached to the skin composed of connective tissue and varying quantities of fat. It is especially thick on the palms of the hands, the back of the neck and the soles of the feet. It serves to anchor the skin onto the underlying tissue. In other areas of the body it is loose and the skin may be freely moved back and forth. Inside the body we have other layers of fascia, which wrap up the organs, muscles ligaments and tendons. They bind things up in parcels keeping them separate from each other. Deep fascia surrounds muscle bellies, holds them together and separates them into functional groups. It also fills the spaces between muscles and, like superficial fascia, carries blood and nerve vessels. To explain in layman's terms: If you can imagine that you have chopped some-ones head off and they are standing upright. If you were to look down at the cross section of the neck without the head what you would see would be circles of fascia that would disappear inside, extending continuously throughout the body from head to toe.

To get a feel of fascia and its relationship with other structures I suggest a simple exercise: Pull up the skin on the back of your hand. Notice how the skin does not pull up entirely (like when you pull a baggy shirt away from your body). This is because the fascia is holding the skin down. If you try this on various parts of the body you will notice how it is easier to lift the skin and fascia but more difficult in other areas. A surgeon will use fascia to stitch bits of our insides back together after we have been operated on. It is very strong.

Fascia is more complex than this little explanation, but it will suffice for the needs of this book. I could go on to explain for example that in the thigh superficial fascia forms a continuous layer over the whole of the thigh and that it consists of areolar tissue containing in its meshes much fat. It may be separated into two or more layers, between which are found the superficial vessels and nerves. I could also tell you that the superficial inguinal lymph glands, the great saphenous nerve, and several smaller vessels separate the two layers from one another.

However, enough of this nonsense!

Fascia is very strong and is made up of collagen fibres. Collagen reminds me of Charlie Duncan who runs a butchers shop in Troon. Charlie has won awards for all sorts of pies and things but it is his pork and chive sausages that I find to be most succulent and agreeable, especially for breakfast on a cold winters morning. Like most butchers Charlie uses artificial collagen for the skins. Collagen is a kind of protein that is the principal constituent of white fibrous connective tissue (as occurs in tendons). Collagen is also found in skin, bone, cartilage and ligaments. It is relatively inelastic but has a high tensile strength. Thus under the skin all of the bits inside us that incorporate the collagen are wrapped in fascia. But how important is fascia in back pain?

Accepting the concept that a muscle is wrapped in fascia we must also understand that the nerves are very close to it. The two things in essence are one. They depend on each other. When we hurt our backs the fascia around the muscle is not happy. It is hurt and reacts by de-hydrating. It becomes dry. This is the reason why sometimes you will see people with back pain who will be bent one way or another. The fascia around the muscle being like a piece of chamois leather that has been left in the sun has shrunk. The muscle fibre has to go with it and thus your body becomes stuck on the one side. In this condition the muscles in surrounding body area become upset. You become upset and you are pained. Of course again using a piece of chamois leather as the example, if you leave it in a bucket of water for half an hour it will re-hydrate. Then it will be relaxed and easy to stretch. The fascia around a muscle reacts in much the same way. Re-hydrated it relaxes and gives the muscle its own space. The fully hydrated muscles allow the skeletal frame to float back to where it should be in your body. The nerves no longer get nipped and the pain disappears. Encouraging the fascia to re-hydrate is one of the merits of the HG that allows the muscles to relax and the body to begin to heal.

There are many muscles in the body: about 400 main muscles that split into 639 named muscles in all. They all have a task to complete. Most of them tend to operate in groups. They don't act on their own. As with most things in the body, we have two of them on each side. The longest muscle in the body is Sartorius. It stretches from just below the bump on the side of your hip, across the front of your thigh until it disappears on the inside of your knee and joins to the top of the tibia. (The tibia is the larger of the two bones, joining the knee to ankle). The largest muscle in the body is Latissimus dorsi, which covers most of the lower part of the back. The smallest muscle, much like the smallest bone, is in the middle ear. These delicate muscles are called stapedius and tensor tympani. They allow the subtle hearing apparatus to move so that we can hear sounds clearly.

In a normal adult, about two fifths of the body weight is muscle. The actual figure depends on the individual. A body builder will weigh more. Teenagers have less, but more forms as your body grows.

However to return to the subject, normal muscle action is a pattern of responses of groups of muscles. In other words muscles have anatomical individuality, but they do not have functional individuality. Thus when we hurt a little muscle or ligament in the back, the other muscles around it recognise this. They go into defensive mode to protect it from any further damage. Our muscles go into spasm. As I explained earlier in the book, this is probably the worst thing that can happen. It is excruciatingly painful. As it has only ever happened in areas of my low back it has made me wonder why.

In the low back there is a virtual absence of bones apart from a few vertebrae. Above the waist, the heart, liver and internal organs are protected by the skeleton. Below the waist, the pelvis protects the reproductive system. Between these two areas we have a mass of soft tissue and lots of muscles. This lack of bones in this area gives us the ability to bend and twist. This I suppose is the reason why I have often stated that the top half of my body is in good condition as is the bottom half, but the hinge in the middle is broken. My back pain has more often than not been located in this vulnerable area.

Of course the skeletal bones between the ribs, the intercostal muscles, rectus abdominus etc, have a job to play in keeping us flexible and stable, but this not where we experience back pain. I suppose that any neurosurgeon, orthopaedist, or chiropractor will tell you that there can be many sources of low back pain. They will tell you that the problem can be caused by a variety of things. It could be vertebrae, invertebral discs or even nerves. X-rays or scans may well give some insight into the back pain problem.

Then the surgeon will be only too delighted to operate, the chiropractor to manipulate. However, they are forgetting the muscles. The soft tissue!

It is my opinion that this is wherefrom all back pain emanates. Yes of course some of us may have a prolapsed or herniated disc. A lesion (bulge) of the disc pressing on the nerve root and yes, the surgeon may well be able to open your back and trim away the offending particle, but are you willing to take the risk? In any case has the surgeon got it right? Just because his teaching suggests that incision into the body is the correct method of repair does not necessarily mean that he is correct. I mentioned in a previous chapter that in America the physicians have developed a method of reducing the bulge on the disc by injecting the centre with an enzyme, which reduces the swelling. What are they using? Pineapple Juice! Injected with a fine needle using miniature camera laser technology to let the surgeon see that he is sticking the needle into the exact spot where it is required. And all of this without the need to open up the back! Sounds a much-improved idea to me! But is there a better way?

My 'Holy Grail' describes a method whereby the muscles in the back, probably in spasm for whatever reason, are asked to return to their original position. In this relaxed position the nerve that is being nipped and sending pain signals will have its own space and will stop sending pain messages. The muscles are encouraged to re-hydrate and relax. This is done by sending a message from a muscle via our feed-back loop system to the brain. The brain of course is a map of the body. Before we are born, in our mother's womb the map of our bodies is perfect in every way. Then we are born (which can be a trauma in itself), lead our life's, go to work, have repetitive strain, play a sport, have an injury, fall from a tree, etc. Gradually a new map grows in front of the original that we were given. The old map is still there but remains hidden behind the new one that has evolved. The HG seems to have to ability to make the new map disappear. This in turn allows the body to heal. The traffic lights in your body that were on red can be turned back to green! In saying this it does seem that God was a cartographer. Everywhere maps abound. There are over thirty different maps concerned with vision alone. Likewise in somatic sensations such as touch and joint and muscle sense there are several maps.

It is perfectly acceptable that when the muscles relax that a herniated disc can slip back to its own source and for the lesion on the disc itself gradually to recover. With the muscles in this stress-free condition the skeletal frame will return to normal. It is especially important for back pain sufferers that the pelvis is in its right place with the muscles connected to it in control without being stressed. The pelvis controls the lifting of the legs, but in doing so it affects the muscles, which are connected to the lumbar spine. All of the muscle groups around this lumbar area are heavily involved in our day-to-day activities. The demands that our bodies make on them are vast. They are thus the chief source of our back pain problems.

Muscles determine the bodies shape. Bones go where the muscles put them. Bones stay where muscles keep them. Thus when considering back pain we should always look at our posture. The way we stand. Some of us walk as if bent like a half shut knife. I see it every day, especially in older folk. The sorts of people who have become accustomed to walking down the road and when they do they look at the pavement. An example is an old lady who came to my clinic last year. She was much stooped and she had low back pain. I gave her a treatment per the 'Holy Grail' and suggested that she should have an appointment with me once a week for four weeks, this being the maximum number of treatments that I will give except in exceptional circumstances. When she came for her third treatment she came into the clinic and said "Mr Steele, I've got my breasts back". I looked at her astonished that an elderly refined woman would say such words.

I smiled. I thought for a moment and then I told her that her breasts had always been there. It was just that her posture had been bad. She had become used to looking at the ground as she walked. The treatment that I gave her improved it and it made her stand up straight. When she did this, the breasts came back up with her, once again a visible part of her anatomy, where they should be. Not swinging around at her waist as they had been. Girls have other problems though.

Little girls because of their charming sweet posture tend to stand with their tummies out. Probably you have noticed it. By doing this they tilt their pelvises forward sticking their bottoms out behind them. Thus girls get into bad habits right from the beginning. Worse though is the problem of wearing high heel shoes. This does the same thing to the pelvis by tilting it to a position that it really does not want to be in. In little girls the wearing of high heeled shoes should be abhorred. The muscles in the hip have to work overtime. The result is that in time to come they will undoubtedly suffer from low back, buttock, and pelvic or sciatic pain. Additionally wear and tear on the hip joint is a possibility with this leading to arthritic conditions and hip replacement surgery. The problems that a woman has at childbirth can often be the result of postural problems as a child/teenager. Too many times I have treated women with sciatic pain that evolved as they give birth to their first child. This is good business for me but in essence could have been so easily avoided.

Parents today are so keen to get braces on their children's teeth to improve the 'posture' of the teeth. They do this not just for cosmetic reasons, but to improve the bite and so on. Why don't they do the same job for their posture is beyond me, Parents are blissfully unaware of the fact that the soft tissues, the muscles, tendons, ligaments and fascia of their children are getting stuck where they just don't want to be. As time goes by when the child grows these tissues tighten down into this unaccustomed position and they end with postural problems.

In later life this postural problem is difficult to resolve. The muscles have become accustomed to being where they shouldn't.

An awful lot of the problems of adults with low back pain are caused by postural misalignments, which have stacked up in their formative years. These misalignments have nothing to do with the skeleton. As I have said the skeleton floats in the 70% of the water that forms the main part of your body. It is the muscles which do the controlling.

The well balanced body of an erect person standing in a comfortable position should be able to have a line drawn through the nose, the breast bone, the middle of the pubic bone and end at a point half way between the feet. A similar line can be drawn on the side, through the ear, shoulder, hip and ankle. Thus it can be shown with the aid of a plumb bob that a person either has or doesn't have proper structural alignment. I have seen this done to patients although I haven't done to any of the folk who come to see me. I am aware of a therapist who has a clinic in Manchester who uses this form of test. Apparently he asks all of his patients to submit to this type of examination. He asks them to stand in some feet prints that are fixed on the floor of his consulting room. Adjacent is the hanging plumb-bob. Then with their permission he takes Polaroid pictures of their posture, both facing front and then to the side. The pictures will show where the plum-bob hangs in relation to the person's structural alignment. Of course in a business such as his it is impossible for the therapists to keep pictures. The patient takes them home with them. He then gives treatment per the HG. After perhaps three sessions he asks the patient to stand on the same foot prints and then he takes more pictures. Then when comparing the original with the new pictures both he and the patient can see just how much correction the body has made. The posture will be better. The back pain will have reduced. The muscles are relaxed, doing the job they were designed to do and will be in the right place. A well-balanced and aligned body! In relation to gravity, that is.

Gravity is something that works against us every day. When we arise in the morning we are half an inch (12.5mm) taller than we were when we went to bed the previous evening. Why is this you may ask? In the chapter about the importance of drinking water, later in the book you will find a fuller explanation; however for the time being let me explain simply that as you sleep the joint capsules between the vertebrae relax. They re-hydrate. Fill up with fluid. Pure water! The lubricant our body relies on. Thus the joint capsules are each that little bit larger. The combination of each little bit on all of the capsules when added together allows that you have this addition to your height. However when our bodies are out of position, out of alignment, the tissues that hold our bodies together, the muscles, have a harder job working against gravity. This is why posture is important to the good health of our muscles and why the muscles are so important to us. In space the body does not experience the downward pull of gravity that it does on earth. As a result the gaps between the spines expand and astronauts do actually get slightly taller. When they get back to Earth of course, things immediately return to normal.

In studying the mechanical action of a muscle, we cannot treat it as a single unit, since different parts of the muscle may have entirely different actions. Nerve impulses control and stimulate different portions of the muscle in succession or at different times. Until a few years ago when I started to study anatomy and physiology or human biology as it is now referred to I would have assumed that each muscle did only one specific task. However as with all things in the human body I have quickly come to accept that every little bit of us is quite a complex piece of machinery. Muscles fall into this category.

Muscles are in a mechanical sense units. The muscle fibres constitute the elementary motor elements. They accept the message from the brain and turn this through the use of energy into action.

In muscles where the fibres run in a straight line from the origin (the bony attachment of the muscle closer to the trunk) to the insertion (the bony attachment which goes through the longest range of movement of the two bones, during the normal action of the muscle), a straight line joining the origin and the insertion will give the direction of the pull. Many muscle names include terms for body locales that tell you the specific origin and insertion of each muscle. In such cases, the first part of the name indicates the origin, the second part the insertion. The genioglossus muscle, for example, originates in the chin (genion) and inserts in the tongue (glossus).

If however, the muscle or its tendon is bent out of a straight line by a bony process or ligament so that it runs over a pulley-like arrangement, the direction of the pull is naturally bent out of line. The direction of pull in such cases is from the middle point of insertion to the middle point of the pulley where the muscle or tendon is bent.

These two examples are just a smidgeon of what goes on in the workings of muscles. I have written this to give you just a little insight into what goes on when you flex your arm. For example – just to raise a cup of tea to your lips takes around 100 muscles to perform the action. Muscles are multifaceted. Their strength depends on many factors; the number of fibres in the cross section: whether the fibres are parallel and have the same direction of the tendon; whether the muscles have coarse or fine fibres and so on. Too complex and involved for discussion in this book! However the point I am trying to make in all of this is that simply stated we couldn't survive without them. At the same time in relation to low back pain, they have a very big part to play.

Please always remember that it takes 43 muscles to frown yet just 17 to smile.

So despite the fact that you frowned when you picked this book off the shelf, thinking that it would be just another load of junk written by a loony who knows nothing about back pain, by the time you have finished reading it and absorbed all the information in it, you might just have changed your opinion. It might just bring a wee smile to the face and take some of the ache and the spasm from your muscles.

Chapter Sixteen

IT'S ALL IN THE MIND

As I sit down to write this chapter it is ten minutes to midnight. I should be in bed. I am tired after a hard days work. Physically I am exhausted. Yet all day the thoughts that I will try to put down on this piece of paper have been swirling around in my head. Thus despite my tiredness I have dragged my fatigued body into my study.

The fact is that the brain is the boss. It runs the show controlling just about everything that you do. It is more powerful and much faster than any computer you've ever used. It is large and in charge – so large that it fills the upper half of your head. Take it out of the head and it looks like a big soft wrinkly lump. How then can something like this control your every movement? It decides whether or not your back pain is going to trouble you today.

How does the brain work?

Lots of people have researched the workings of the brain. The answers written down would take millions of pages to write. Throughout the centuries there have been an awful lot of people interested in how it works. Despite this, there are many things that we still don't know about it. Having said that here is some information that I can give you:

- An average brain weighs about 3lbs.

- It contains about 100 billion nerve cells. (1,000,000,000,000 neurons). About the same number of stars that exist in the Milky Way.

- Each nerve cell has between 1000 and 10,000 connections with other nerve cells.

- None of these connections are in any way dormant, but not all of the connections are in use at any one time.

- The percentage of the brain in action at any one time depends on what we are doing.

After the age of 20 the brain looses about 1 gram of its weight per year as nerve cells die and are not replaced. Older people, those over 70, can still function properly despite losing so many cells over the years. This means that some of the brain cells must be able to double up on what they have to achieve for us. However the complex nature of the brain means that those of you out there who are trying to clone a human being have a hell of a long way to go before you will be able to. Heart transplants are fine. Brain transplants? I don't see it in my lifetime.

To put this into perspective, let us look at medicine and where it is today. Doctors know more or less what to do when most parts of your body go wrong. That is, with the exception of the brain. In brain science we are still in the dark ages. The knowledge that scientists have in relation to learning about the brain is at about the level of the total medical knowledge of the times when Florence Nightingale (the lady with the lamp) was alive and working at the field hospital in the Crimean War (1854-56). If you consider the steps that man has made in his understanding of medicine and how much things in general medicine have developed since Florence, then you might just begin to realise how far we have to go in explaining the workings of the human brain.

I have no doubt that quite a few neuroscientists will have dug around in the brain of some poor unfortunate trying to find answers. Why do we laugh? Why do we cry? As a baby in the cradle, how do you recognise your mother? As a man on the way home from the pub (with perhaps more alcoholic beverage inside you than is good for you), how do your find your way home? Are you on automatic pilot? Why do we dream? What is consciousness? No matter the digging I have no doubt that the scientists come up with but a few of the answers. Despite perhaps a couple of hundred years of research they have yet to come up with the answers to even the simplest of questions. The biggest revolution yet to come: understanding ourselves.

The strangest thing about all of this is that we have evolved from the ape or so we are told. The brain that the ape had has evolved into what we have today. How did this happen? How have we managed to progress to the extent that we are able to do all sorts of wonderful things. Type the words in this book even. Strange indeed! Yet there are even bigger questions to answer. How on earth can this evolved brain manage to ask questions about itself? How can it ask questions about its own existence? Who are we? Where did we come from? What happens after we die? I think the point that I am trying to make here is that there is an awfully long way to go in understanding the human brain. A lot of exciting things have still to happen in the neuroscience world. It lags a long way behind general medicine. If I were today to be given a chance to get into medicine and in particular the neuroscience branch I don't think that I would have a moment's hesitation. I would find it exceedingly exciting to be at the cutting edge of a science that has baffled us for so long.

Apart from back pain my BNT is able to help many things. Included is Multiple sclerosis. MS has many diverse symptoms. Thus a study of my BNT in relation to MS, to prove the efficacy, would be difficult. However I have recently made an application for some funding for research that may give us some answers to how my therapy seems to have some effect. With regard to the brain and MS it would seem to me that there may be a tremendous redundancy of connections in the normal adult brain. Like reserve troops they are called into action only when needed. Sadly by losing the myelin sheath on the nerves that carry the messages to the muscles in someone suffering with MS, much like a burst water pipe, the message just doesn't get there. The feed-back loop is broken as is the connection from the brain to the muscle that it wants to activate.

The brain region is responsible for smooth, coordinated swinging of the arms when we walk. This swinging is different from the one that controls gesturing and indeed is activated by a different part of the brain.

To answer this we need to look at the anatomy and physiology of the motor and sensory systems of the human brain. Consider what happens when you or I close our eyes and gesticulate. Despite our eyes being closed we still have a vivid sense of our body and the position of our limbs. To create this body image at any given instant our brain combines information from many sources: the muscles, joints and motor command centres. A truly remarkable happening yet we don't have much idea how the brain is able to do all this. Of course on this point there is probably some scientist in another part of the world who has just discovered how all of this works. Thus I stand to be corrected.

What we do know is that every time a command is sent from the brain to the motor area of a muscle, they move. At the same time the message is sent to two other major processing areas of the brain (cerebellum and parietal lobes) informing them of the intended action. Once the command signals are sent to the muscles, a feedback loop is set in motion. Having a command to move the muscles execute the move. In turn signals from the muscle spindles and joints are sent back up to the brain, via the spinal cord, informing the brain that "yes, the command is being performed correctly". These two structures help you compare your actual performance with your intention. I just wish that this would happen when I swing my golf club.

At my clinic I have treated a number of people that have suffered from a stroke. This is a terrible thing to happen to anyone and I have been pleased to help with their recovery. None of what I do in this is evidence based and certainly demands yet another study. However I find that I am able to help none the less. When I studied the words that I could find that are written about what happens to the brain in stroke situations I found that some people who have stroke have a form of learned paralysis.

What actually happens is that when a blood vessel supplying the brain gets clogged, the fibres that extend from the front part of the brain and down the spinal cord are deprived of oxygen and sustain damage, leaving the arm paralysed. But in the early stages of stroke, the brain swells, temporarily causing some of the nerves to die off but leaving others simply stunned and off-line. During this time when the arm is non-functional, the brain receives a 'visual' feedback that tells it that the arm is not moving. After the swelling subsides it is possible that the patient's brain is stuck with a form of learned paralysis. A temporary form of illusion of non-movement! Some BNT seems to be able to help in the recovery and movement returns but as I have stated before we start making any false claims about this, it needs further study such that it can be examined in greater detail and in bigger numbers of patients.

When we experience back pain, special pathways in the brain are activated simultaneously both to carry the sensation and to amplify it or dampen it down as needed. Known as 'gate control' it allows us to modulate our responses to pain in answer to changing demands. This might explain why some of us are able to sit in the dentist's chair and have him drill holes in our teeth without the need for anaesthesia and perhaps why acupuncture works for some of us and not others, or indeed why some women can give birth and don't experience pain during labour.

Pain is susceptible to the placebo effect (the power of suggestion). My BNT has no negative side effects, but from time to time a patient may experience some flu-like symptoms for a day or so after. That is why I never tell a patient what may or may not happen after a treatment. In other words - If I were to tell a patient that he or she will feel terrible the next day, by the use of placebo there is no doubt that some of them will feel just so. What we have to appreciate here is that pain is an illusion – constructed entirely in your brain like any other sensory experience.

The opposite can be described as the feeling that one gets in orgasm when love making, when a wonderful feeling of all-round goodness courses through the body.

With regard however to back pain management, in a way like emotional freedom technique, I would like to carry out an experiment of which I have heard similar versions from different sources around the world. In essence the body image that we have and I suppose the pain signals that we get with it could be changed with a few tricks. For example: get a dummy rubber hand that you can find in a joke shop. Place it on a table in front of you. Put one of your hands behind you and place your own hand matching the dummy behind a curtain. Next have a friend stroke the dummy hand and your own hand at the same time. Have your friend do this in such a way that you cannot see the body movement that they will make stroking your hand. In a few moments you will experience sensation as if it is coming from the false hand. The first time that I did this I found weird. I knew full-well that it was a imitation hand in front of me but despite this I couldn't get the thought from my head that indeed it is was a dummy hand in front of me and that there should be no sensation coming from it. I have yet to work out how to convert this into helping back pain but watch this space!

The autonomic nervous system (ANS) has much to do with our responses to faces, objects, situations that we have to deal with on a daily basis. The ANS controls all of our involuntary actions. We blink, salivate, and digest our food. Our heart beats, yet in all of these actions we have little if any control. The brain is the command post that operates without us or indeed despite us. Thus when we put food into our mouths it disappears in our own chemical factory to appear at the other end as something totally different. We give no regard to what happens in the factory nor do we to the pace of or heart-beat that will automatically speed up as we run up stairs or indeed slow down when we go to bed at night. However there is another side to this.

When we are emotionally aroused by a sexually alluring partner or indeed threatened by a menacing person – this information travels to the face recognition part of the brain (the control centre for the ANS), which in turn using our nerve fibres sends messages to the muscles, heart and other parts of the brain and indeed other parts of the body preparing it to take appropriate action in answer to what we are confronted with. Then we are in a well-know situation known as 'fight or flight'. In an instant your brain makes a decision and tells your body what to do. In the process the heart-rate will rise as will the blood pressure. You will also start to sweat, not only to dissipate the heat that is now being generated in your muscles but also to give you a better grip of the weapon that you are holding to bash the fellow who is about to punch you or indeed a better hold of the branch of the tree that you are going to grasp as part of your escape route. Damp skin has been used for a long time as the indicator in lie detection machines. Sweaty palms are part of emotional response.

However, leaving aside what we do know about the brain, it would appear that in general medicine many of the important matters that affect us have already been developed. Some months ago I watched a television programme about a man in America. He had been given a mechanical heart. The man knew that he did not have long to live. He had other complications with his health, which will mean that even with the new heart or not, he will die anyway. However, the point is that he is a decent fellow. He has donated his body to science while he is still alive and allowed it to be experimented with. This though mirrors the work of Professor Christiaan Barnard from South Africa who pioneered heart transplants.

I seem to remember that his first patient did not live all that long. But look how far we have come since then. Heart transplants are the norm. People given them these days live for lots of years.

Despite this it will, I am sure, take us quite some time before we are able to offer spare-part surgery for back pain allowing for the complexities of the spine, the nervous system and all that is combined in this special place. Heart transplants are crucial to our survival. Back pain isn't.

It is of course possible that spare part surgery for most bits of our bodies will happen in time. Indeed I am sure that we are well on the way. Of course some bits may take a bit more work than others. The liver and the kidneys have a very complex bit of work to do in our bodies, yet in hospital patients are linked to machinery which is able to clean the blood and so on, much as our own bodies do. With modern technology I am sure that someone will come up with a miniature machine, which will fit inside your body, replacing the part that has worn out, gone bust. On the other hand, how long will it take to replicate the human brain?

The brain you are given at birth is what you have to live with for the rest of your life. At birth we have all the nerve cells we are going to live with. An adult brain is four times the size of a baby's. However, as we grow, the number of cells that we have don't increase, it is just the size of the ones that we already have that do. The foods that we eat are the healthy diet the brain needs to develop. Protein for growth and carbohydrates for fuel!

I understand that in infancy it is best to have your brain stimulated. (Exercise for the brain cells). The sooner that your parents start, the better! Babies left alone have been found to take longer to develop than ones who weren't. In later life of course it is better to take care of your brain. My mother always told me that too much alcohol was bad for the brain. Destroyed the cells, she said. I think that there must be a grain of truth there.

The brain makes up about one-fiftieth of the body's weight and is protected by the skull. The brain receives signals from inside and outside the body. It controls all of our basic functions such as heart beat, temperature control, salivation, food digestion and so on. We don't have much control over any of this. As previously explained the brain uses the autonomic nervous system to send the signals to the bits of our bodies that perform these tasks. The brain also allows us to decide what we want to do next, like walking and running. In addition it allows us to complete more complex tasks like writing a book such as this. Of course it also controls our moods and emotions. Much like my pain and anguish when my back muscles were in spasm!

The cells that make up the bones and skin grow constantly to allow wounds to heal and bones to knit. However, nerves in the brain and spinal cord cannot do this. Scientists are trying to find out how to make nerve cells grow such that some people who have suffered spinal injuries might regain some of their movement; however research is still at a very early stage. Thus these poor souls remain wheelchair bound because their damaged nerves cannot grow back. When I was attending my doctor with my back problems, he told me to prepare for life in a wheelchair. Indeed, I had come to terms with what he told me. His words and the consequential thoughts that I had were the catalyst for this book. I just had to share all of this with someone, in the hope that they may be able to benefit from my retrospection.

However I am very grateful that my back problem as it has turned out, was muscular rather than damaged nerves. As they say, there is always someone worse off than you are out there in the big world. This is probably the reason why I have never moaned too much about my back problems and the pain that it gave me, no matter how excruciating it may be.

The nervous system that I mentioned above is part of what controls your every movement. Apart from the autonomic system, which controls our involuntary actions we have sensory nerves, which take messages to the brain and motor nerves, which take the signals from the brain to the part of the body that you want to move. Energy is the transmitter of these signals. Energy travels two and a half times round the world per second. This is why if you touch the point of your nose with your finger you can feel it instantaneously. In this action two things had to happen: a message went from the nose to the brain to say that it is being touched and a signal went back from the nose to the brain agreeing that it did. As it happens so quickly, it feels instantaneous.

Another example of this would be in the kitchen when a person involuntarily touches a hot plate on a cooker. It seems that instantly the persons hand lifts from the hot surface. However this is not the whole story. As the persons hand moved towards the hot plate the motor nerves were telling the muscles to do so. At the same time if we were able to slow down the actions of the arm and hand we would see that the sensory nerves are already picking up the message that the hand was heading for a very hot place and that the body would be burned. At the speed of 300 metres per second the energy in us sends these messages up and down the feedback loop system. The brain takes a fraction of a second (a long time in reality) to work out what is going to happen, to stop the motor nerves from doing the action of placing the hand on the hot plate and to set the whole motion in reverse. Sensory and motor nerves working in harmony with the brain then prevent a serious burn. How the brain manages to do this of course is a mystery to me, but again I stand corrected if some wise owl who reads this book can enlighten me. Suffice to say that it is just another wonderful thing that the brain is able to do for us.

Understanding how the brain works is indeed a complex subject. I will not go on too long about it, but I do feel that if you can comprehend how your mind works, then it might help you to get to grips with your own general malaises and back pains. Nonetheless the nervous system in our bodies is itself complex. It is a network of millions of long thin cells called nerve cells. Different types of nerve cells do different things. Receptor cells pick up the messages from the outside world. They carry this information to the brain. The brain decides what action to take and sends the signal back to effecter cells. Muscles are effecter cells.

The brain itself has various sections that have specific tasks to complete.

Sensory information goes to the thalamus, which stores early responses. The thalamus is the junction box. The cerebellum is where the muscle movement is programmed. It is though badly affected by alcohol. Hence the reason why a drunk man staggers about! The cerebellum is not in control of the muscle function. The cerebellum is also where things are programmed and committed to memory. In childhood you touch a hot surface. It hurts. Mother tells you not to do it. You remember and don't do it again. The cerebellum doing its job! Learning the piano and where all the keys are is another example.

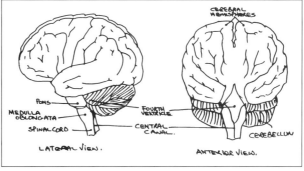
Side view and rear view of the brain.

Writing this book I have to have some kind of idea where the letters are on the keyboard. Not all that long ago I could not type a word. My wife tried to teach me the 'quertyoip' method of touch-typing. She wrote all of the keys onto a piece of paper the same size and shape as the keyboard and sellotaped it on top. I then had to place my hands under the paper and try to touch type. I could not do it! We fell out! Stupidly I argued with her and shouted at her because of my inability. She left me to my own devices. I started with the keyboard placed to the right and typed with one finger. But this was very slow and eventually the finger ached from overuse. So I had a think and decided that I would place the keyboard in front of me. I then started to type with two fingers and two thumbs. Eventually I got the hang of things and the brain took over guiding the fingers to where it remembers the keys are although in doing so I hardly look at the keyboard. Thus I am self-taught. The cerebellum guides my fingers! It remembers where every key is and has worked out where to place fingers as I type.

The brain anatomy is controlled primarily by the thalamus. It controls our mood. We can be hyper–anxious, over motivated. Our adrenalin and cortisole production will be high. Our heart rate and blood pressure will be up. Our hunger metabolism, immune system and libido will be down graded. Our overriding sympathies will be 'fight or flight'. On the other we may be hypo –parasympathetic. Babies do it. They switch off and go to sleep. Remarkably a cat on the operating table in general anaesthetic can go into parasympathetic mode. Switch off and die. Vets have to be very careful. The opposite of fight and flight in a hypo situation is that we will probably pee or soil ourselves.

The pathway in the brain works much in line with the following: Let us imagine that we are walking along a path in the jungle. We see a snake. The thalamus receives the signal that is a snake. We are instantly stimulated. The amygdala triggers a fast reaction (run for it – fight or flight). But a clear image of the snake is sent to the conscious brain for a considered response. This considered response sends the signal that in fact it is not a snake at all. Indeed it was a twig. We breathe a sigh of relief and continue our journey. The brain as you can see is a complex item. In understanding it you may realise how much control it has over the muscles in your back which have just gone into spasm.

Finally in this chapter on the brain let me tell you a story. It has nothing to do with my bad back but a lot to do with brain.

On the 18th February 1995 I attended the rugby match at Parc Des Princes in Paris where Scotland were to take on the mighty French team.

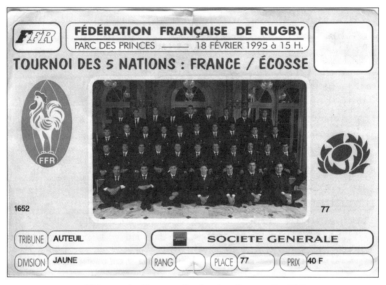

Ticket to the France v Scotland rugby match 1995

I had completed ten years as a committee member at Kilmarnock Rugby Football Club. In 1992 I was proud to be elected President and asked to serve in the position for two years. In all of the years on committee I attended most, if not all, of the international rugby matches in the Five Nations championship (Scotland/England/Ireland/Wales/France). The match against the French was held in Paris. Despite the fact that I had been to Paris several times I had never witnessed a Scottish victory. In reality we had not won on French soil for twenty-five years. However with hope in my heart and with my good friend Jack Whyte we set off once again more in hope, than in certainty of a victory! The blessing, apart from the rugby, was the solace of copious amounts of good French food and great French wine to drown our sorrows if, as expected, we again lost the match.

Parc de Prince is on the south side of the city. A giant concrete structure it is the home of Paris St Germain, a football side. However, with true French hospitality they gave up the ground whenever the rugby matches came around. It was a smashing place to visit with great viewing. The seating was very near to the pitch. You could just about touch the players. I do remember Jack telling me not to eat the hamburgers that were being sold in various mobile booths at the side of the road on the way to the stadium. I often laugh when I remember him telling me that they were made from the remains of some old dead camel that had been hanging in a warehouse for weeks before. Salmonella and all sorts of horrible digestive things come to mind. However his words of wisdom saved me from hospitalisation - or worse.

The match was exciting. It flowed from end to end. We scored first. Then the French levelled. And so it continued in un-abating nail biting exhilaration. No one sat. We stood throughout the match. We shouted. In a tribal manner we sang our Scottish songs until we were hoarse. We were hyper. With just a minute to go the French were leading.

Then Gavin Hastings, the Scottish fullback collected a kick from the French who were trying to pin us in our own half. Gavin grabbed the ball with both hands. He surged into overdrive and ran at the opposition. Passing player after player we gasped as he approached the far touchline. Avoiding one last desperate French tackle he dived over the line and touched the ball down. We had scored. The points were level. However the job was not complete. We had to win the match. Gavin had to covert his touchdown by kicking the ball between the posts.

Hearts in mouth we crossed fingers, toes and about every part that the body would allow. Gavin had some deep breaths. Taking a few steps back he stopped and composed himself. The brain reminded us that he had missed kicks like this in front of the posts before now. We prayed. He ran at the ball and kicked it. It flew skywards right between the posts and at the same time we screamed in delight. The match was over. For the first time in twenty-five years we had won on French soil.

But then to our amazement the referee turned to the centre circle indicating that in fact it was not time up. The match had not ended. Oh Lord how were we going to stand the pain? The French had some really good players in their team, such as the great Serge Blanco. Many of them were world-class. Someone like him would surely seize on an opportunity like this and conjure a score from nothing despite the fact that there were but seconds of the match left to play. Without doubt we were worried that we were to be denied our bit of glory. We prayed. The referee whistled and once again the match surged into life. Tired legs and bad backs had to grind into action.

I don't know how many extra minutes the referee played after Gavin had scored but it seemed an eternity. How our gallant defence repelled the efforts of the valiant French forwards is beyond me. Yet for that little eternity they did. Then the referee blew his whistle to end the match. We had won.

The joy was immense. We hugged and kissed. Man to man in true Gallic style. Our faces hurt with the smiles, which would take a long time to fade.

The players left the field of play. The Scots euphoric! The French devastated. We waited and shouted for our brave lads to reappear from the dressing room. After a while they did come back onto the field, much to our pleasure. Socks around the ankles, they strolled across the battered turf towards the waiting fans. We bowed in exultation to their glorious victory. Much later we left the ground. Before though, we had a beer or two and a glass of wine. Drinking alcohol at a match in France is allowed. Much more civilised than we are in Britain. Thus we set off for our hotel. A good wash and shave and we were off for a great night of celebration.

The French and the Scots have a great affinity. The 'Auld Alliance': A friendship that goes back to the times of Charles Edward Stewart (Bonnie Prince Charlie). Thus as we stepped out into the cool Paris evening air we were greeted by gracious Frenchmen and women who congratulated us on our epic victory. And so with Jack by my side we set off in more or less a straight line for a fine restaurant where he had thoughtfully reserved a table. The menu was of course in French. It did though look exciting and not wishing to show my lack of understanding of the finer points of the French language I ordered my food.

I cannot remember what we started with. I could not care. I think that it was something deliciously fishy? We were by now deep into our first bottle of finest Pouilly Fume. In any case the food was phantasmagorical. I was enjoying my evening. In what by now was blurred speech, Jack and I were having a discussion in probably too loud a voice about the exquisiteness of the stunning women around us in the restaurant.

After a mid course of Crème de menthe water ice, the main course arrived. Jack had more fish. I had something in pastry. With relish I attacked it. I sawed off a big portion and bit into it. I munched away happily. The headwaiter came over and asked if everything was in order. We were effusive in our congratulations of the excellence of the culinary staff in his kitchen. I sawed off another portion and started to chew again. This time a bit of my intelligence, my subconscious knocked on the back door of my by now befuddled head and suggested that all was not well. What I was consuming did not just taste or feel in the mouth like any food that I had ever eaten before. Now don't get me wrong. I like oysters. I enjoy the salty taste and the slippery texture. I swallow them with relish. However this was a different texture altogether!

I turned the plate around to examine the pastry or more to the point the contents of the gastronomic delight that I was paying a fortune for. Suddenly realising what I was eating I stood from the table. I made a beeline for the nearest exit. It led down a staff corridor to a back door to the restaurant. I ran at the far wall in the courtyard. My stomach exploded and I vomited the contents onto the ground before me. I felt awful. I had sobered up in the quickest time ever.

It took me quite a few minutes to recover my senses. A kindly waiter tapped me on the shoulder. Noting that I was Scottish and assuming that I had simply consumed too much alcohol he proffered a damp cloth to wipe away the remains from my face. The cool wet flannel was just what I needed. Dusted down I returned to my place in the restaurant. I did not eat any more food that night. I did though put away a consummate amount of alcohol to drown the thought of what I had consumed, wrapped in pastry. What was it by the way? Oh it was calves brain!

Chapter Seventeen

LIFTING, SITTING, STANDING, SLEEPING etc.

On a daily basis those of us with bad backs, have to take care with every movement we make with our bodies. Nonetheless we all have lives to lead. In this we have chores that we must try to accomplish in one-way or another. Much of this is dull, yet mundane things like dressing, shopping, and going to work and so on, all have a risk of one kind or another. And so we must take care. The problem is that we don't. In the years prior to BNT I would have periods when I would be debilitated with severe back pain. Then I would go though a period of recovery. And then I would drift into a period where I would be comfortable and pain free. I would forget about the last time that my back muscles were in spasm.

In this relaxed state I would take chances. I would get into bad habits. Then – Bingo! It would happen again. Attempting something stupid like trying to move the sofa in the lounge and the spasm would return. Yes of course I had moved it lots of times. But then I was younger and fitter. Then it would seem that I was in the condition where I was older but no wiser. However the sofa had to be moved. I had not cleaned under it for weeks. It could not wait until Sheila got home from her shopping trip. And so I would stupidly attempt the task on my own, never giving a thought to whether or not my back would stand the strain.

When Sheila eventually arrived home from shopping, there I was on the floor. In agony, I was immobile. With my back muscles screaming in pain I was afraid to move. Of course when she opened the door to find me once again in this position she was not surprised. She had seen it all before. Nonetheless I did feel stupid.

What made matters worse was that I had to admit that I had been attempting a task that could have waited till she came home. With two people to lift and move the sofa it would have been a simple task. There would have been little risk of muscle spasm if I had waited for her to assist me. But I was a man – a stupid one it would seem.

There are today more people who live alone. In this day and age the numbers grow. Lot's of us for whatever reason it would seem enjoy our own company. Nevertheless those of us who live on our own still have to move sofa's unaided. And so accepting that there are different categories the common denominator is that no matter whether we are married or single we will all attempt stupid things that will endanger our backs. Thus I have written this chapter in the hope that by applying a little bit of common sense to every-day chores you will irrevocably change your life style. In reality I don't think you have a choice.

Back pain is an affliction, which affects about 80% of the population in Western countries. Sadly the indications are that it would seem to be on the increase. In Victorian times manual labour was part of life. Bad backs it would seem did not exist. At least the documentation from those times does not record it as such. Today we have all sorts of mechanical aids to help us. Despite this back pain is more prevalent. Why is this?

Let us go back in time. What did our ancestors do? They climbed trees. They chased wild animals. They dug the ground and cultivated their food. They made their own tools. They chopped wood and lifted and carried it to their primitive homes. At home they had no furniture. They squatted or sat on the floor. They were mobile and active. Thus the mobility in all of the joints was maintained. Their muscles were stronger and were used for what they were intended for.

In today's modern world we have failed to adapt. Back pain in essence is something of the western world. Aborigines in Australia and tribes in Africa have a very low incidence of slipped disc. The very fact that they have to use their muscles to do the jobs that we use mechanical tools for gives them the reward of greater physical fitness and mobility, and freedom from back pain.

The spine is made up of a column of bones called vertebrae. The skull is at the top. The pelvis is at the bottom. The human backbone is made up of 33 vertebrae. There are 7 cervical vertebrae in the neck. Under this we have 12 thoracic vertebrae each carrying a pair of ribs. Then we have 5 vertebrae in the portion of the lower back (lumbar spine). The next five are fused to form the sacrum (between the hips) and the lowest 4 form the coccyx, which a long time ago was our tail. The vertebrae have cushions (discs) between them, which act as shock absorbers. The discs need to be hydrated by drinking regular amounts of plain water. (See chapter on the importance of drinking water). At the back of the spine the vertebrae are held to together with ligaments: small sections of relatively non-elastic condensations of fibrous tissue, usually joining two bones in close approximation. Of course the spine is strengthened and made moveable by groups of muscles. This structure changes your back from a rigid rod to a moveable spine.

The spine carries the weight of the top half of the body. The spine includes a spinal canal, which is the protective channel for the spinal chord. The chord is of course connected directly to the brain. The cord is also connected to the nerves between each vertebrae and these control the movement of the trunk.

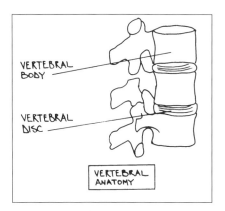

Discs cushioned between the vertebrae bound by ligaments and muscles allow movement and flexibility. Without discs the spine would be like a bit of steel rod. We would be stiff and straight and would not be able to bend in all of the directions that the spine allows us to. As I explained in an earlier chapter the portion of the body in the middle (for lack of a better medical description) the bit, which has the tummy at the front, has nothing to protect the spine other than the muscles which surround it. However, while this vulnerable area gives us the ability to bend, it is also the bit that we have to look after when we are bending or lifting things, playing golf or indeed any sport.

Backache is not always caused by something being wrong with your back. It may well be lumbago (strained muscles) or strained ligaments. Either of these is easily damaged if you are not fit or indeed if you attempt something simple but do so stupidly. An example of this would be a woman emptying her shopping trolley at the supermarket. The damage occurs when the woman arrives at the car to unload the trolley and reload the heavy bags into the boot of her car. She stands facing the trolley, with feet planted. She lifts two bags of groceries at a time and turns to face the boot of the car, without moving her feet. At this point the spine is twisted. Worse, though, she is about to subject it to an extreme bending movement converting the 30kg load (15kg in each bag) to a strain of approx 100kg on the spine. Then she stands up straight and grimaces. Of course by that time the damage is done. The muscles are strained.

Women suffer back strain by constantly having to work over a low sink, leaning across a bed to tuck the bedclothes in, or bathing and lifting the baby from the bath. I could give hundreds of examples where men will hurt the back in an industrial injury. Men though in my opinion are stupid. Too brave for their own good!

They seldom admit that they have back pain until it virtually cripples them. The discs injured in this type of strain are those between the lumbar vertebrae. The thoracic vertebrae are so well supported rigidly by the ribs that their discs are unlikely to be strained. But the cervical discs are commonly damaged by faulty posture, ageing allowing the head to sag and of course by whiplash in a car accident. This can be the cause of pain and tingling in the hand or arm and perhaps the cause of pain higher up in the shoulder blades.

Such pains are sometimes called fibrositis: a vague but ill-defined pain in and around muscles. Faulty posture (which could affect either the backbone or the muscles where the pain would appear to be) is an important factor in bringing on attacks. Sitting in an awkward position, or sitting tensely in any position can start the pain.

Tension, in turn has many causes, including all kinds of anxiety. In treating this disorder, relaxed and mechanically efficient posture generally does more good than aspirin and massage. Thankfully the therapy that I practice is able to address not just the physical but also the emotional side of things that can often be the cause of stress and tension.

Thus we have a number of things that must become part of our daily lives if we want to lead a life without back pain. Simply stated we have no choice. So in an effort to help you, I have described a number of sketches and instructions, which you should commit to memory and have them, become part of your life, for the rest of your life.

POSTURE:

(A) STANDING. The chapter about the Holy Grail will help you understand that we can improve how we do this. The body has the ability. However to help it we should try to walk tall, all of the time. Head up, with shoulders in a natural position should be the norm. Shoulders should be neither too far forward nor back. Standing like a sergeant major with the shoulders back is bad as is the opposite with shoulders hunched forward when the ribs squeeze onto the pericardium (the space around the heart). Bad posture may not cause any discomfort, but continual poor posture will in the long-term cause back pain. Good posture will help prevent back pain. Thankfully the BNT improves structural alignment.

Gravity works on us all day long. Thus the sensible thing to do is to try and have a posture such that the centre line of gravity goes through the middle of our bodies. If we allow our bodies to slouch over the centre line, then there is a greater pull of gravity on the body and more stress and strain on the back muscles.

The hollow that you have at the bottom of the back is called a lordosis. Earlier I mentioned the Aborigines and other African tribes who don't have furniture to sit on. They sit on the ground or they squat. In consequence they have a much shallower lordosis than we have in the Western world and of course less back pain.

All sorts of people come to my clinic in Glasgow in the west of Scotland. Confidentiality is absolute. However allowing that you will never know to whom I refer I have a story to tell that is appropriate to this chapter.

A relatively elderly lady came for treatment for her back pain. I gave her a consultation as I would normally. Explained in detail what I would do and then proceeded with the first course of the therapy. A week went by before she came for her next visit. She came into the clinic and as I worked with her she told me that she was a keen gardener. We swapped stories about horticulture, not that I know much about the subject. She was happy that we were making progress and that her back pain was receding. Another week later she returned for her third treatment. Again in conversation about her garden she told me her neighbour was as keen as she was to produce a splendid array of colourful flowers and to make this last through the summer. She could see what her neighbour had in her front garden but she had always been curious to know what she grew in her back garden. That was until this week when she noticed that for some strange reason she was an inch or so taller and now that she could see over the top of the wall between her and her neighbour she was able to satisfy her curiosity.

I smiled as she told me the story. Then I explained that the therapy had managed to do for her was to improve her structural alignment, and make her stand straight. The lady was surprised but happy that she could now understand this phenomenon.

She realised and now accepted that the gardening work that she spent so much time had allowed that she stooped lower and yet lower as the years progressed. She had become used to it and thought that it was the norm. Now after just two treatments she could see that her body had worked in harmony with the therapy that I had administered.

Now she walks tall. Well, all 4ft 11ins of her!

If you stand at work it is important firstly to think of your posture. Try to educate your body to put the lordosis into the spine. When you stand though, the blood in the arteries and veins stagnates. There is not a lot pumping it around the system and eventually it can lead to varicose veins. Thus I suggest that every twenty minutes or so you should complete the knee lift exercise as previously explained. Commence standing with both feet on the floor. If you can, hold onto the wall, a door handle or something adjacent. Gently raise the left knee as far as you can without forcing. Put the foot back onto the floor. Raise the right knee in the same way and allow the foot to drop back to the floor. Repeat this ten times on each side. As you complete the exercise you will see that gradually the knees will rise higher and a little higher each time as the muscles are encouraged to stretch. If you do the exercise quickly you will hurt the muscles and make them work against you. Take time. Done properly you should begin to feel a warm glow in the groin as the revitalised blood and energy begins to course through the lower part of your body. At the same time you will be pumping the lymphatics, which cleanse the blood. Your heart will thank you for it.

If you are a woman and walk a lot, please wear sensible shoes. High heels are bad for backs.

(B) SITTING. Always choose a chair that is comfortable, one that supports your back. If it doesn't keep a couple of cushions handy to stuff in behind the lordosis.

It is important that both feet should be flat on the floor, not dangling in front of you. Women should NEVER sit with their legs crossed. This pulls the pelvis out of position and cuts off the blood supply to the lower limbs. Always sit back in the chair. Don't slouch. If you slouch there is every possibility that in addition to back pain you will have a chance of aching neck and shoulders and headaches.

Sitting too long in one position (as the sketch showing bad posture – opposite) is just one of a number of positions that will make back pain worse.

One thing that you must NEVER do is to be fooled into purchasing a back support: a belt that wraps around your waist and buckles at the front. I have seen all sorts of examples as they are advertised regularly in the press. Some have all sorts of gadgets built in that purport to offer one benefit or another. My suggestion would be throw it in the bin if you have one. By wearing such an

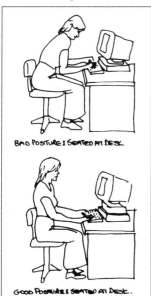

BAD POSTURE : SEATED AT DESK.

GOOD POSTURE : SEATED AT DESK.

accoutrement you are doing your body no favours. The belt may give a comfortable feeling that it is protecting and helping you. In actual fact you are allowing the belt to do the work of your muscles.

Using such an implement over a long period of time will allow the muscles to waste and in turn your back will get weaker. I get angry when I see the adverts for this sort of thing especially when they are suggesting that they are particularly helpful when lifting or carrying loads or playing sports. This is simply not true. This kind of advice leads you down a path to dependency on the belt and in time back pain ruin. Of course you may say that you have seen weight lifters using them in competition; however the belt is only on for a short time, not all day. In addition weight lifters avoid strain by keeping their backs straight, squatting and then using the muscles in the legs to take the strain and do the lifting.

I had the occasion a couple of years ago to approach a senior football club in Scotland. I read in the press that the captain of the club had had to end to his playing career. The stories told that his back muscles were in continuous painful spasm. The club had tried all sorts of remedies to return the player back to full health. In desperation they had sent him to see some eminent specialist located in Harley Street in London. In the process they had spent quite a few thousands of pounds. All their efforts had been in vain. The player's career as far as they were concerned was over. He had been a good player in his time. He was going to be missed.

I telephoned the club and spoke with the manager. I suggested that my therapy may perhaps help return the player to full health. It was agreed that I should meet with the player, his physiotherapist and the club doctor. If looks could kill I could see that from the expression on their faces that they did not believe a word that I had told them in explanation as to how this therapy works. Even more strange was the work that I did to the player. They were totally unconvinced. However, reminding them that they had tried all sorts of lotions, potions and bone crunchers without success, I explained that my therapy takes a little time for it to work and asked that they allow me a week or two to prove a point.

I told them that the body will heal when it is able. In some of us I can find a more or less instant response, while in others it can take quite a few days to kick in. We parted with the agreement that we would re-convene at the same time a week later. I crossed my fingers.

My therapy does not have 100% success. Nothing does. However the success rate is high. Generally I would expect 75% with the treatment of back pain having greater success. It was no surprise to me when we met the player the following week to find that indeed his back pain had improved. The muscle spasms as I fully expected had ceased. His mobility had improved. The club doctor and physiotherapist were still sceptical. I administered more treatment and taught my back pain routine.

Needless to say in a few short weeks the player started walking and then jogging before he finally returned to playing football. Regaining his place in the team, his colleagues were pleased to see him and had much to ask about the strange therapy that he had received. The result was that at the Monday morning clinic at the football club I became a popular person. In time I was treating 20 or so players every Monday.

Unfortunately politics abound at football clubs such as this. Despite the status of the club in the Scottish Football league the club was in financial difficulty. The management didn't pay the players. They didn't pay their suppliers. They didn't pay me. Eventually the manager led a revolution. Pay the players or they wouldn't play football was his ultimatum. The club paid up, but in the course of events that followed there was a takeover by a new regime. The new board sacked the manager. I was also asked to leave. Despite the fact that I received no recompense for my efforts, I was satisfied that I had been able to prove a point. My therapy had helped when all else had failed.

For those of you who work in an office, please have a look at your workstation. It is of equal importance that the desk and computer should be at sensible height. Most of these things are adjustable today. Fiddle with the height adjusters until everything is at a comfortable level. If your feet don't reach the floor, put a box or a couple of books under until they rest comfortably on top.

In the office it is possible that you will be able to adjust the angle of the seat such that your knees are below the hips. If you are not able to have such a chair or indeed if you do a lot of work at home, as more and more of us seem to do these days, it is possible to purchase a wedge of foam which can sit on your existing chair. This improves your posture and reduces the risk of back pain.

BENDING AND LIFTING

There have been many articles/books written on the subject. Indeed Governmental departments issue guidelines. How many of us though pay a blind bit of notice? Until of course when it is too late and the damage has been done. If you have a bad back, and have something that gives you a bit of grief now and again, be it wear and tear or whatever, then I would urge you to give the following words your careful consideration. As far as I can see more than a third of all over-three-day injuries reported each year to the Health and Safety Executive are caused by manual handling injuries. Lifting, supporting and transporting of loads by hand or bodily force is the culprit. The cost to employers in the UK is somewhere in the region of £500 million pounds and growing.

Many manual injuries build up over a period of time rather than being caused by a single handling incident. Comparing this with my own problems, I would say that this is a true statement. No single incident caused my problem. Indeed, I admit that I cannot actually remember when I had the first bit of trouble.

However, most manual handling injuries occur when people are engaged in work at factories, offices, warehouses, farms, building sites and such like and in such places are asked to lift things that they shouldn't. It is important that employers should consider the risks from manual handling and give their employees as much help and information about the subject that they can. However, too few seem to do. Most of us - the employees - are left to fend for ourselves. Thus if you are in this category I would ask you to consider the following:

AVOID: The need for hazardous manual handling, as far as reasonably practical.

ASSESS: The risk of injury from any hazardous manual than cannot be avoided.

REDUCE: the risk of injury from hazardous manual as far as reasonably practical.

TAKE CARE: to use the proper equipment provided for safety.

INFORM: Your employer of any activities that you would consider a risk of injury.

PROVIDE: Mechanical aids wherever possible. Even a simple sack barrow can make all the difference, never mind the improved productivity that your employer can benefit from.

GOOD HANDLING TECHNIQUE: Before I attempt to lift anything I always adopt the following principles.

1. Stop and think. How heavy is the load to be lifted? Do I need help to lift it? Are there any obstructions?

2. Position the feet. Always stand with the feet one in front of the other.

3. Adopt a good posture. Remember that the muscles

in the legs are strong. They are able to take to take the strain. Thus these are the muscles we will use when lifting. However we can only do this if the back is straight.

4. Get a firm grip. Try to keep the arms within the boundary of the legs. If you can keep the load close to the body. Cuddle it!

5. Don't jerk. Lift smoothly. Take a deep breath before you start and exhale as you lift.

6. Move the feet. Don't twist the trunk when holding a load. Shuffle the feet round until you are facing where you want to deposit the load.

7. Put the load down slowly and carefully. If necessary put it down and then slide it into the desired position.

Lifting in the home can be just as hazardous for the housewife. I would ask every housewife to adopt the following simple routine when lifting anything, no matter how simple or heavy it may be. I am blessed with a good woman who is happy do most of the housework. However, as a back pain sufferer I have damaged myself by bending to lift a handkerchief.

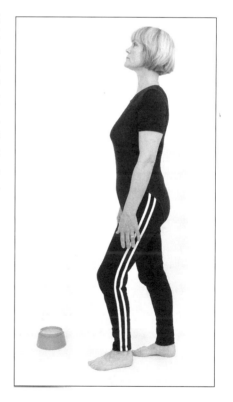

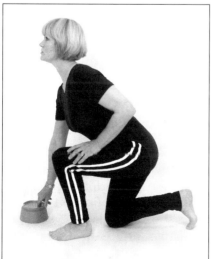

Look up. Reach out and place a hand on the wall to steady things. Place one foot in front of the other.

Use the leg muscles to take the strain. Drop down onto one knee.

Slowly bend forward and pick up the item to be lifted. Hold the item resting the hand on the knees. Readjust the feet, and look up.

Stand up once again using the muscles in the legs to do all of the lifting. If you have done all of this correctly you should be able to rise vertically just like an elevator. The centre of gravity will be through your head and down through the middle of your body.

GETTING IN AND OUT OF A CAR.

I often look in amazement at people getting out of a car. They open the door. Then in a rather unladylike manner they swing one leg out of the car and then the other. The main part of the body is left facing front. The knees are hardly together. The back is twisted. In this silly position we attempt to stand and haul ourselves out of the car. Arriving at a standing position I have never been surprised to see a grimace on the face. A sure sign that some damage has been perpetrated in the lumbar spine region and that at least some muscles have as a result gone into spasm.

In a world where 'the car is king' we don't walk as much as we should. We spend most of our lives hopping in and out of vehicles of one kind or the other.

And of course when we are pain free, we think that we can get away with anything. Thus I find that most folk get out of a car in this fashion. In the process they risk tearing the fibres of the small ligaments that hold the sacroiliac joints at the rear of the pelvis. Without getting too technical I will try to explain why this happens.

The pelvis (pelvic girdle) consists of two hipbones at either side and the sacrum and coccyx at the rear. The hips form a sort of round shape with our spine fitting into a slot at the back and the femur (the big bone in the top of the leg) fitting into a socket underneath on either side. The femur is the longest, heaviest and strongest bone in the body. All of the bones of the hips are connected to other bones; however the portion that takes the strain, if you swing one leg out at a time, as you get out of a car is the sacrum. The sacrum (the base of the spine) is closely connected to the ilium (hip bone) on either side with ligament. Ligament is virtually non-elastic. If you open your legs as you swim the breaststroke there is no pressure on the joint, the water is supporting your body. However people who are careless when getting out of a car swinging their legs open put a lot of pressure on the sacroiliac joints when they attempt to stand first on one leg and then the other. More often that not the result is that some of the small fibres in the ligament get torn and you then have consequential back pain. So my advice when getting in and out of a car is to keep the knees together.

DRIVING A CAR: Sit in a comfortable position with the spine sunk well back into the seat. Hold the hands out in front with the hands higher than the elbows. Drop the shoulders. Keep the occiput open – Eh? The occipital bone sometimes called the 'bump of knowledge' is the back of the floor of the skull. It forms a moveable joint with the backbone. The brain stem passes through a large hole in the occipital bone to become the spinal cord. If you are little and need to peer over the top of the steering wheel as you drive the car you will undoubtedly have to look upwards.

This reduces the flow of blood and nutrients to the brain. Thus when driving, try to adopt a position that will allow you to look at the road ahead, but with the head focusing slightly below the horizontal. Of course it is important to check that the driving seat is upright and that you can reach the pedals comfortably. Don't drive for too long a time. Stop every so often. Get out of the car and walk around a bit. Do some knee lifts and windmills (as previously explained)

WALK TALL: Always keep an upright posture. (A few sessions with therapy from me or from others that you can find in the web pages attached will help this). Keep your back straight and shoulders square. Keep your shoulders relaxed and loose. Avoid sudden movements.

BE A GOOD CHAIR PERSON: Sit in straight backed chairs. If you must sit on a sofa, make sure that your spine is supported with lots of cushions. Stuff them into the small of the back. Relax but sit upright. Don't slump in sofas. Don't sit twisted at a table. Never cross your legs as you sit. Apart from anything else if you cross the legs as you sit you are cutting off the blood supply to the lower limbs.

GARDENING WITHOUT MISERY: Digging the garden for me is out of the question. However I do like to potter around doing a bit of weeding at times. Thus I have searched for gardening tools with long handles to save me from bending. I never spend more than 20 minutes or so, on each job. Taking debris to the compost heap I only ever half fill the wheelbarrow. I keep the load to the front of the wheelbarrow such that when I lift the weight is over the wheel.

WEIGHT CONTROL: Being overweight puts an awful lot of strain on the weight carrying joints, especially those in the spine. This will also increase the curve of the spine (lordosis) but more to the point will increase the rate of wear and tear on the joints, which of course are more or less irreplaceable.

Being overweight means that you probably don't exercise and

not exercising means that you won't be fit. Thus you are more likely to suffer from back pain.

PUTTING TROUSERS ON: How many times have you heard of a man who hurt his back trying to put on his trousers? Men are stupid when it comes to things like this. I see it often. Standing out in the middle of the floor with one leg in the trouser, they hover in an un-balanced state while they attempt to shove the other leg into the bit of the trousers they are holding. More often than not they miss the opening for the leg. Get tangled in the trousers overbalance and fall to the floor. The damage to the back – well who knows? However all of this could be avoided by simply leaning an elbow against the wall. It stabilises the whole body and makes the task simple. Anyone with a dodgy back should adopt this sensible method. Women should do likewise.

Chapter Eighteen

EXERCISES

Before starting an exercise routine I would advise that you have a word with your GP. Tell him what your intentions are and have him give you a good check over before commencing with anything strenuous. Let us have his approval for you to commence. Keep in touch as you get fitter and always go with his advice.

I have no doubt that exercises are good for a bad (weak) back. Years ago, the considered opinion of the medical fraternity was that lying on the floor for long periods was the best route to recovery from back pain. If you were unfortunate enough to be admitted to hospital for an operation on your back, or indeed any part of your anatomy, you could expect to be away from your family for an extended period. I can remember a friend going to hospital to have his appendix removed. A relatively simple procedure! He was kept in for a week after the operation. Today we know better and accept that staying mobile is the answer. The day after an operation for hip replacement patients are encouraged to get out of bed to stand and walk a few paces up and down. A few days later they are discharged. Not many years ago they would have been bed-ridden for weeks. Recovery was slow! Now we know better. The same applies to anyone suffering with back pain.

Exercises for the back should be carried out in a slow and controlled fashion, starting with just a few repetitions of each exercise session and gradually increasing over some days until the required numbers of repetitions are reached. It is of extreme importance to ensure that you don't take risks. Thus apart from walking which in itself should be risk-free, all of the other exercises that I teach are done on the floor or on a bed. Flat on your back you should not be able to do much damage.

Of course being overweight complicates a back problem, in that all the excess weight on the abdomen has to be supported by the muscles in this region, and in turn the lumbar vertebrae. However by adopting even a simple walking routine, as part of your daily activities, should help you to lose weight, which in turn will strengthen the muscles in the lumbar spine and in time will allow you to recover something resembling full health.

I have heard people talk about diet and the fact that they lost just two pounds in weight. Two pounds seems such a trifling amount they will say, especially when considered in relation to the amount of physical effort expended when trying to achieve weight loss. Whenever I hear this from a patient I will ask them to carry a two pound bag of sugar (or two pound weight of any kind) in their hand for a couple of hours. You can see the relief in the face when they put the weight down. Then they begin to see just how important it is to the body to lose even a pound a week if you are overweight.

WALKING:

I would encourage anyone with back pain to walk every day. If your back is in a mess and you are reading this book in bed or on the floor, my advice is to get mobile. Inactivity is bad as this allows the muscles to become lethargic, de-oxygenated and flaccid. Muscle has memory. If you allow your back muscles to remain in a static state for long periods, then the body will assume that this is the norm. When of course you attempt to move, the body resists, invariably a muscle or group of muscles gets pulled, the nerve adjacent gets restricted and you get pain. I can think back to the days when my muscles would often be in painful spasm because of this. I spent long times lying on a bed, on the sofa or on the floor recovering from yet another painful muscle spasm. I would be afraid to budge, as I knew that one wrong movement would set the whole thing off again. I am no coward, however, the resulting pain was simply too much to consider. Thus I remained static for long periods.

Simply getting up from the sofa and having a wander around my house would have made all the difference. Today, of course I know that I was a stupid person. I accept that being active is not only the route to along and healthy life, but additionally and crucially a recipe for success if you suffer with back pain.

My advice would be to commence with little bits of walks here and there. Begin with a stroll around your own home. It may surprise you just how many routes that you can find from the kitchen to the bedroom, along the hall into the bathroom and back again. A few minutes at a time are sufficient. Then take a rest. Once you have regained your courage, then it is time to attempt to walk to the end of the street and back. Repeat the walk as many times a day as possible. As the days go on gradually increase the distance you travel until you can walk without pain and do so for

30 minutes. The aim is that you should build up the pace at which you walk, such that eventually you will be able to walk quickly. My regime takes me out of the house five times a week. Winter and summer, good weather and bad, it makes no difference. I am happy to get out in the fresh air. I always carry a bottle of water with me and sip from it at regular intervals as I walk. I will speak about the importance of drinking water in a later chapter; however for the time being accept the fact that it is important. The combination of walking and drinking water lubricates the joints and keeps you supple. Of course the benefit to the cardiovascular system is tremendous. Your general health should improve and with the entire oxygen intake you will sleep better at night.

Thus the first and best exercise there is, is walking. The benefit of course is that it is free. It costs nothing to walk. I live in a nice town. I vary my route depending on the time of year, the weather conditions and so. However I enjoy walking. It has become part of my life. I fully understand the benefits. I purchased one of those little portable radios with earphones that are unobtrusive when popped into my ear lobe.

They allow me to hear the traffic noises such that I won't get knocked down as I cross a street, while at the same time permit me to listen to my favourite classical music as I walk. I have a number of routes that I use and have developed as time has gone by. Initially after getting a little bit of fitness I found a route that was two miles in length. To find how long it was I simply drove my car around the circuit and recorded the distance. Today it takes just twenty minutes to walk the circuit, which tells me that I am walking at a pace of six miles per hour. On a Sunday, when I have a bit more time for leisure activity I have a route that takes me on a round trip of about ten miles. It has taken my time to build to this level of activity. Thus my advice to anyone recovering from a painful back is to take things easy in the beginning and only gradually over a period of time increase the distance that you travel.

I am obviously now walking more quickly and thus must be fitter, but it was not always so. When I first started walking at a faster pace I noticed that I was breathing quite heavily as I walked and when I had completed the route, it took a time for me to recover. Invariably, I would sit in the car, while I would sweat profusely. At the same time I could feel my heart beating quickly. The reason for this is that the muscles had built up lactic acid (anaerobic respiration). Every cell in the body (and we have millions) needs oxygen to break down the glucose we produce from the food we eat. The glucose feeds the cells to produce energy.

However in the absence of sufficient oxygen, lactic acid is produced. It is however a reversible reaction and the lactic acid will disappear when the oxygen debt has been repaid. We may have to breathe heavily to do this at the end of a brisk walk. As we gradually become fitter, the body becomes more efficient and in turn we breathe less heavily. Then when we walk fast the heart speeds up to pump the required blood and nutrients to the muscles. As we get into a rhythm the heart slows down a bit but the pressure is kept on it which is good for us.

Old age is no barrier to this form of exercise. My father is 93 years of age and enjoys good health. As a child I can remember that he would go for a walk every day. He also drank lots of water. Simple stuff from the tap! We didn't have bottled water in those days. I can still remember that every time he went into the kitchen, he would go to the tap and have a drink of water.

In those days there were no books nor information to let us know that drinking water on a regular basis was good for us, yet without any prompting my father would do this frequently. In hindsight I can see that during his working life, as he toiled in the hot engine-room of the ships that he worked on, that drinking water just became a necessary part of his life. The habit has remained with him and thus, here is he today a happy and healthy chap, both mentally and physically. Even at his age he still goes out for his daily walk, of a couple of miles, no matter the extremes of the weather.

Assuming that you want to get out onto the streets, along the beach or into the park to follow this healthy walking regime there are a number of steps that you should take first as I have said, please speak to your doctor. Get him to give you a check over, to confirm that there is no reason to prevent you from exercising as I have suggested. Next, a visit to your local BNT therapist should resolve any remaining muscle spasm, tone up your body, and set you in the right direction. After treatment you should be given some exercises (similar I would hope to those that I have explained here in the book) that will help to relax the muscles, to strengthen your back and to help set the pelvis in the correct position. The exercises are best done in bed in the morning before you rise, before you are weight bearing, and again at night before you go to sleep. The pelvic toning exercise is one that I learned from the Bowen Therapy Academy of Australia. I don't know if Tom Bowen left us this legacy. Suffice to say that I was taught it in my student days.

I don't think that Tom would be unhappy for me to pass on this little bit of knowledge.

Some of the other exercises are ones that I have learned from my trips around the world or a result of conclusions that I have come to myself. Of course with all of the exercising and walking it will be hoped that you will lose a pound or two. Energy use is based on weight over distance. Thus it doesn't matter whether you run a mile or walk a mile you will use the same number of calories.

It used to hurt me mentally, when I was out on one of my walks, only to be overtaken by two ladies who would sprint past me at an alarming rate. One was a fairly thin and lightweight sort of person. The other was a rather larger lady. Knowing what I do now, I am able to understand that my form of exercise was in the long term better for me than the exercise that the women were in the habit of undertaking. By walking rather than running, I should have less damage to the joints in my body, in that they have less to cope with the jarring than that experienced by the women.

Walking of course is excellent in that the Soleus muscle (mid point between the knee and ankle – at the back of the leg) where it works as a venous pump. I am sure that many of you will have watched a military parade and wondered why the guard who has been standing to attention, suddenly and for no apparent reason faints and falls over. The inactivity by standing on the spot for a long period allows that the blood pools in the lower limbs. The brain becomes starved of oxygen and basically shuts down. The Soleus muscle as it is positioned is activated as you walk. In turn this major pumping action returns the blood from the lower extremities, and back to the heart. In essence the Soleus is the body's second heart. The simple act of tensing and relaxing the Soleus muscle as the guard stood to attention may well have prevented the oxygen starvation.

If by exercise you are able to lose a few pounds, then the resultant weight loss should in turn help reduce your blood pressure.

Clinically speaking I am no expert in this field. Nonetheless from the many medical journals and such that I have read, I am sure that this statement is correct.

THE BREATHING EXERCISE

Before we commence with any sort of exercise it is important to be able to breathe properly. Back pain, headaches, raised blood pressure; indigestion, sweating, palpitations, irritability and anxiety are all linked to one common factor – Stress.

When we are stressed, we won't breathe properly, indeed we may find it impossible.

Stress is a normal physical reaction to an internal or external pressure that is placed on your system. The body then becomes flooded with stress hormones, making the heart pump faster, the breathing rate increases, and the muscles tense up. How often have you been stuck in a traffic jam, late for a meeting? You know the feeling. The pressure builds inside you and some or all of the symptoms as noted above manifest themselves. Stress is a killer. It can be caused not just by the trauma of the traffic jam but additionally by financial hardship, marital issues, deadlines, indeed a whole host of things that affect us on a more-or-less daily basis. Internal pressure (emotional symptoms, feeling tense, brooding, worrying, depression) are all examples of our own inability to cope with these issues and all exacerbate the problem. Many people today suffer from the effects. Some of us use a crutch in an effort to alleviate the problem, such as drugs, alcohol, caffeine, nicotine or sugar. In this there is no logic, in that these chemical substances simply deplete the body of energy, which in turn simply causes yet more stress.

When I was ill with my own back pain, I was often stressed. At the time I didn't know or understand how to cope with the problem. However over the years I have come to terms with the issue and with this experience would offer this advice.

Eat well.

Get physical.

Use your own mental exercises.

I have written a little about good eating in a later chapter and I have explained a bit about how important exercise is not just for people, suffering with back pain. I can also see that talking to a family member or a close friend can be surprisingly effective in helping a problem. 'A problem shared is a problem halved' and all that. However, you may be surprised to find that the doctor who listens patiently to your problems may well have troubles that are yet worse than your own. Thus I would ask you to consider my form of mental exercise, which itself is part of the breathing exercise that I have evolved.

I suggest that everyone should find time on a daily basis, to go through this routine; indeed it would be my opinion that this simple exercise could be life-saving or at least life-extending. There are many benefits. It will relax the Psoas muscles, which in turn relaxes other muscles in the abdomen, diaphragm and chest. Muscles are chums. Thus I find that if you can encourage a group of muscles to relax, then in turn the muscles adjacent will respond and also relax. Settling down the muscles in the abdomen will in turn calm a rather important muscle in the body – the heart. Indeed four eminent doctors wrote an article in the Lancet a couple of years ago where they told of the results of their research that had shown that people who work through this sort of breathing exercise for 25 minutes a week (5 minutes a day) can reduce their own blood pressure by 10%.

However, before we go into the intricacies of the exercise, let me tell you tale.

Some years ago, a lady came to me for treatment. She had lumbar spine (lower back) pain. I looked forward to helping her symptoms, and was very positive in my intentions. I gave her the first treatment. She returned to the clinic a week later. I asked if she had found any improvement in her back pain. She told me that she did not. I explained that 'the man who did the miracles' died two thousand years ago and that sometimes it takes a bit more effort and time before the body will start to repair itself. I administered a second treatment.

When the woman came for her third treatment a further week later (allowing that I usually ask a new patient to have four treatments, at intervals of one week, with a single follow-up a month later), I again asked if there had been any improvement in her pain. Once more she told me no. I was puzzled. I asked her to sit down in my office and we began to chat. At the time I was a relatively new practitioner and was still finding my way, especially with matters other than the physical subjects I had been taught. I had a hunch that this woman was not emotionally stable. I was proved correct, when she told me that she was going through a divorce. In splitting from her husband, she had sorted all of the financial matters without trouble. They had sold the big house, split the cash in the bank and other items of value without difficulty.

The problem between them was that she wanted the family dog and the cherished record collection, and so did he. They had nearly come to blows over this silly subject. It was of course all the more ridiculous when considering that the house they had sold was worth hundreds of thousands of pounds and that in the process they had agreed to split the resulting finances perfectly amicably. The dog and the records were worth little. Yet here they were at loggerheads.

The woman was emotionally a wreck. She started to weep as she told me her story. I did my best to comfort her and after she had regained her composure, I began to explain the fact that her body had to be in control emotionally before it could heal physically. The treatment that I was giving her, was being sucked up by the emotional-side of things. This in turn left nothing to repair the physical side. We agreed that we would alter the treatment, to address the emotional side of things.

The following week when the woman returned to my clinic, I asked the obvious questions to find that not only did she feel better emotionally but her back pain had in addition receded.

In the process of treating the woman, I taught her this breathing exercise, and at the same time explained the reasons why it was important. The exercise is thus:

Find a comfortable position on a bed or on the floor. Raise the knees. Place the feet shoulder width apart. Put the hands on the tummy. Close the eyes. Take a long slow breath in and fill the lungs to capacity. Stop 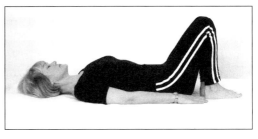 and don't breathe for a second or two. Then, exhale pushing the last bit of air out of the lungs.

When you breathe to fill, or empty your lungs and you stop for a second or two, the lungs will yell at you to breathe. They don't like the idea of stopping. It is after all a natural thing for the body to do – inhale and exhale. It does it all day every day. We just take it for granted.

The body by screaming at the brain, asking it to give instruction to the lungs to breathe will be trying to control the brain. Yet by stopping for a few seconds, you will be instructing your brain to get-a-grip and show that it is in control. The brain will tell the lungs when to breathe, rather than the other way round. By controlling your breath, you will take the first step, perhaps for a long time, when you will be in control of your physical-self.

In the process of taking these deep breaths, I imagine that I am breathing in a good thought and breathing out a bad thought. At the same time, in an effort to fully ring-fence the brain I ask it to do yet one more thing, I ask it to count. Thus as you breathe the words that you should say to yourself should be as follows:

Good thought in, one –stop.
Bad thought out, two – stop.
Good thought in, three – stop.

And repeat, until you have completed thirty breaths in and thirty out. If you get half way through the exercise and lose track of which number you are at, go back to the beginning and start again. If you get twice, half way through then you will have done well.

Allowing that we take about seven or so breaths per minute, it will take five minutes or so to complete the whole exercise. In completing a relatively simple routine we will take the body away from the stresses of the day, rid ourselves of our negative thoughts, calm the muscles, slow the heart rate and ready us for a good nights sleep (doing the exercise before bed time) or setting our bodies up for the rigours of the day that is ahead of us, if we go through the routine in the morning.

As you breathe, it is of course your own choice as to what a good thought and a bad thought you think of. My good thought is my Guardian Angel, who is up above on a big white cloud, high above me, looking after me every minute of the day and night.

I keep talking about – 'she', so I suppose that it must be a woman? Thus as I breathe in, my sub-conscious imagines a big white cloud floating down towards me, bringing all of the goodness that my God and my Guardian Angel gives. When breathing out, if for example I have a headache I would imagine that I am blowing black smoke out of the hole in my head where it hurts. If I had back ache, I would imagine that I was blowing the same black smoke out of a hole in my back, again at the spot where it hurt.

The woman who was going through her divorce breathed in the same good thought as I did, but when breathing out she thought of the man who was soon to be her ex-husband. He was standing at the front door, of her house – right in her face. As she blew out, the black smoke pushed him a little down the garden path. Each time she breathed she was able to blow him a bit further away. When I spoke with her when she returned to the clinic the next week she told me that by completing the breathing exercise regularly she had blown him so far away, that she could no longer see him. Additionally, the dog, and the record collection, that she had fought so hard to retain had become matters of little consequence. After all, a dog would be a hindrance in her quest for a new man and the record collection was so much out of date it was not worth having.

I use this exercise in bed every night as a tool to help me get to sleep. I place my hands on my tummy and take deep breaths in and out. As I write these words I am yawning as my body thinks that I am about to put it to sleep. It has become accustomed to my stress-free life. With practice I hope that you find the many benefits that I have found from this simple, yet so-effective breathing exercise.

PSOAS EXERCISE:

In the process of describing the breathing exercise, I indicated other benefits. One such is that it will help the Psoas muscles to become calm. The Psoas muscles are important to your structural alignment and can prevent you from standing straight. Many a time I have walked down the street in Glasgow and come across a man or woman walking towards me, head up, yet with the top half of their body tilted forward, the Psoas muscles are tight.

The Psoas muscles are the bedrock in a balanced, well organised body. With two on each side of the body they are massive muscles, approximately 16 inches long, that directly link the ribcage and trunk with the legs. Each Psoas is a multi-joint muscle, attaching to six joints and passing over two. It can contract as well as stretch and lengthen. The Psoas is basically a hip flexor. It supports the free swing of the leg in walking, and plays an important part in transferring the weight through the trunk into the legs and feet. It is a guide-wire that stabilises the spine.

Exercises like sit-ups and push-ups not only weaken the Psoas muscle, causing it to tense and shorten, but also provokes additional stress to an already strained back.

People who complain of unilateral Psoas problems invariably run their hands vertically up and down the spine; those who run the hands horizontally across the low back have a bilateral problem. Pain will be worse when the patient tries to stand upright. A frequent addition will be pain in the front on the thigh. Additionally patients will have difficulty when arising from a deep-seated chair. Without getting too complex, problems of this nature can affect bowel movement.

Thus, as you can imagine this is a simple exercise that addresses all of these difficulties may be useful.

The Psoas major and Psoas minor muscles attach to the lumbar vertebrae, down into the pelvis and yet further down to the femur (thigh bone). These muscles are important in the control of pain and have a major influence in the pain-free or otherwise life of someone who suffers with back pain.

The problem that I have with this exercise that it is a simple routine, yet people that I teach it to, don't, in many cases believe just how good it is for them. It doesn't hurt. It is illogical. Most folk that have back problems invariably expect exercises that will hurt, or at least stretch-off the muscles that they think are causing the problem. The common words that I have heard often are "no-pain, no-gain" but simply stated this is not true. My opinion is never to antagonise the antagonist. Thus it is often the situation that I will work around the muscle in spasm without actually putting my fingers on it. The same applies to this exercise. Address this muscle group, give them a bit a TLC and watch what happens. Your body will respond by allowing your structural posture to re-align and let you perhaps for a long-time to stand up straight. The old adage, 'bones will go where muscles put them' cannot be truer in this instance. The exercise is thus:

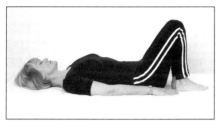

(1) Take the same simple and safe position that I teach in most exercise – on your back – on a bed or a floor. Place the hands by your side. Take some big long slow breaths in and then out, each time filling and emptying the capacity of the lungs.

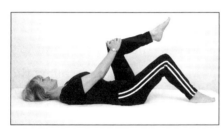

(2) Then, once again inhale. Then exhale, and while doing so, draw the left knee towards you. Hold it with your hands. If you find this impossible, Take a towel and twist it into a rope. Hold an end of the towel in each hand and use it as a lasso to hoop it over the knee. Then using the towel pull towards you (as you exhale).

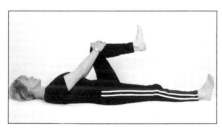

(3) While still holding the left knee take a deep breath, in. Then as you exhale, while again still holding the left knee, allow the right leg to straighten. As you do this, try to point your right heel, such that it stretches as far away from you as possible.

(4) With the legs and pelvic floor muscles held in this position, take another breath in, and then out. Then return the knees back to the starting point as shown on position (1). Repeat the exercise ten times alternately on each side. Only pull the knee towards the chest as far as it will go comfortably.

HIP-SWING EXERCISE:

As part of a routine for people that suffer with back pain, I would suggest that it is best to start with the breathing exercise, then proceed with the Psoas exercise and finally follow it up with these hip-swings.

(1) First take a position on a bed or on the floor (as per position 1 in the Psoas exercise). However this time place the hands behind the back of the head. Raise the knees and keep them together. Keep both heels together.

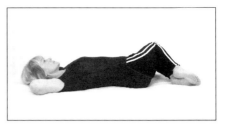

Take a deep breath in, and then as you exhale allow the legs to fall to the left side (as in the photograph).Make sure that the knees and both heels are still together. The right heel as you can see has lifted from the bed. Keeping both knees and both heels together, hold this position for ten seconds. Initially when you allow the legs to fall to the side you will find that the muscles in your back will become tense. They may hurt a little. Talk to them. Tell them to relax. You may be surprised to note that in taking a few deep breaths in and out, at the same time subconsciously talking to the muscles that are hurting will in fact help them to relax.

(2) Take a breath and return the knees to the starting point.

(3) Breathe in, and then as you again exhale, this time allow the legs to fall to the right side. Again hold for ten seconds or so before returning once again to the starting point.

(4) Repeat the exercise to either side for 3 repetitions.

PELVIC TONING EXERCISE:

This exercise is again an old yoga exercise that I learned years ago (and also taught me by the Bowen Therapy Academy of Australia). That Tom Bowen had a good opinion of it is gratifying. It is as it says a simple pelvic toning exercise.

As with all of the exercises that I have described in this book, the golden rule is - if it hurts, don't do it. Send me an e-mail (through my web-page) or phone the clinic, where I will be more than happy to answer any queries. The exercise is thus:

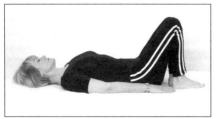

(1) Lie on your back. Have both feet flat on the bed. Pull the knees up such that the feet are near the buttocks.

At the clinic I would carry out a simple test to find which side of the pelvis would be tenderer (if any). However on the basis that you can't do the test on your own I am sure that you will realise which side of your body hurts, has a dull ache, or just feels that little bit more uncomfortable. Assuming that the more tender side is the right, commence the exercise with the left side. (2) Raise and straighten the leg as far as it will go until the knee is locked. Don't pull it with your hands. Use the muscles in the leg to take it up as far as it will go.

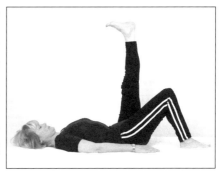

(3) Gently lower the straightened leg to the bed. Doing this as slowly as you can, you are making the pelvic muscle work against the weight of the leg.

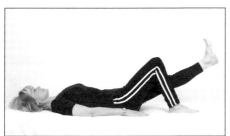

(4) Slowly drag the heel of the leg you have just lowered along the bed, up towards the buttocks, and back to the starting position.

(5) Repeat the exercise with the other leg.

(6) Repeat the exercise on both legs for 10 repetitions.

It may be that when you start this exercise that after one or two repetitions you are exhausted. This is fair enough. If it is really exhausting commence with just a few repetitions and gradually as the days go on increase the number of repetitions that you can manage. The golden rule of any exercise is that you should never work through the pain. If this exercise hurts, don't do it. Talk to your therapist or your doctor. You may have wear and tear in the hip that requires someone qualified to have a look at it and give advice. When in doubt –ask!

HAMSTRING EXERCISE:

Bad backs are often accompanied with tight hamstrings. There are three muscles in the hamstring group. The muscles are at the back of each leg, stretching from the hip to behind the knee. The muscles are strong hip extensors and knee flexors. All three of the muscles tilt the pelvis posteriorly and two of them rotate the hip. Thus if they are tight they can imbalance the hip which in turn can effect the position of the spine. At all times they should be soft and supple.

The term 'hamstring' originated in eighteenth century England.

Butchers would display pig carcasses in their shop windows by hanging them from the long tendons at the back of the knee. I just wish by the way, that the England cricket team would listen to what I have to say about this exercise. I have often watched them out on the pitch, prior to a match starting, bending and stretching the hamstring muscles as far as they can but never giving a thought to relaxing them off after.

They don't seem to know that there are two parts to the exercise.

The following is a simple exercise to gently stretch the hamstrings. It could be done easily in the changing room prior to a match.

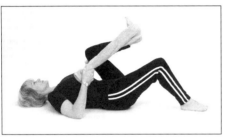

(1) Lay on the floor or on a comfortable bed with both knees raised. Roll up a towel to make a rope (or use a trouser belt). Hook the towel over the left foot.

(2) Pull the towel towards you and at the same time straighten the leg as best as possible. (3) While in this position, take a breath in and then as you exhale, gently pull on the towel to tighten the hamstrings at the back of the leg. Don't pull with excess force, such that it hurts. (4) Relax the leg a little. (5) Take a deep breath in and then on the exhale repeat the stretching

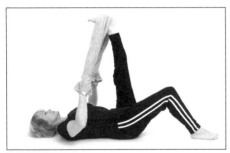

exercise again. (6) Repeat the exercise, each time attempting to stretch the muscles just that little bit further. When you exhale and tug on the towel, talk to the muscles. Tell them to relax. You will be amazed what your body will do when you tell it to do something. Allow your brain to be in control of your body rather than as with most folks, the body rules the brain.

The secret in any exercise is again never to work through the pain. Thus don't pull until it hurts. If an exercise starts to hurt, back off a little. If you give your body a chance and encourage it without hurting it you will find that it will respond by indeed stretching just a little bit further each time. When I attempt this exercise I look at a mark on the ceiling where my foot would point to the first time that I pull it towards me. Then and each time I pull, I would try to go just a little further. Of course there is a limit to how far the muscles will stretch.

Repeat this hamstring exercise by applying six pulls on each leg. It is best done night and morning (if you have the time) for a week or two or until the hamstrings feel soft, supple and gently stretched to capacity.

After completing the hamstring stretches, stand up and do some knee lifts on each leg. The reason for this that we are playing two antagonists off against each other: the hamstrings at the back of the leg and the quadriceps at the front.

This is the principle of alternately stretching and using a muscle (and is of course the last thing that you will see the England cricket team doing.)

ABDOMINAL STRETCHING:

When you get to the point that your back is becoming pain free it is time to start thinking of some abdominal strengthening exercises. Again we will do the exercises in bed in the morning before arising. It is best if the exercise is done after the pelvic exercise, with the two exercises becoming part of a routine. There are no photographs with this exercise. However it is a simple that I hope you will understand.

(a) Lie on your back with your knees bent up and feet flat on the bed. Place your hands at your side, palms down.

(b) Gently lift the hips from the surface of the bed to a comfortable position, but no more than two or three inches from the bed.

(c) Then uncurl the spine from between the shoulders down to the hips. Think of each individual vertebra landing on the surface of the bed as the spine unfurls. Repeat the exercise as many as you can manage pain free.

BACK STRENGTHENING:

(1) Lie flat on the floor, face down, with a small pillow under your abdomen. Place your hands folded under your forehead. Keeping the leg straight, raise the left leg about six inches from the floor and hold this position for a count of five. Return to the starting position. Repeat ten times on each leg or do as many repeats as you can manage without pain.

(2) Lie flat on the floor, face down. Place the hands by your side. Take a deep breath in. Then exhale, pushing as much air out of the lungs as you can manage. At the same time pull the muscles in the tummy into the abdomen, sucking them up as far as you can manage. Without breathing, hold this position for ten seconds.

(3) Relax the muscles and take a few breaths in and out. Then repeat the exhale and tummy tucking exercise as many times as you can manage. If at first when you commence with this exercise and you find that after just two or three repetitions the stomach muscles ache, then stop. You have done enough. If you are serious about getting rid of your back pain problems you will find that continuous use of this good exercise will allow you to build to ten repetitions fairly quickly.

The advantage of this exercise is that there is no danger as you will do all of the work flat on the bed or floor.

More importantly by strengthening the tummy muscles you will in turn help your back muscles to cope better.

EXERCISE FOR OFFICE WORKERS:

In the office we are pretty static. We sit on the hamstrings. We reduce the flow of blood and nutrients to the lower limbs. The body becomes lethargic. The brain slows. We don't think quickly. As a result you can often look round the office to see someone yawning in the middle of the day. It should not happen. In Japan as I have explained, in most offices, they have a routine that takes just a couple of minutes, yet is repeated on the hour every hour to revitalise every bit of their bodies. My exercise (in two parts) is one that any person who sits or stands for long periods should adopt and repeat regularly throughout the day. It is an exercise I teach to all of my patients, including the doctors and surgeons that attend my clinic.

This two-part simple exercise for office workers or indeed anyone who has to sit around for long periods is known as 'knee-lifts and windmills'. Together they will invigorate and waken up a tired and lethargic body, especially if you work in a hot and stuffy office and even more so if you work at a PC for long periods. Stepping away from your desk for the few minutes it takes to go though this routine is worth the effort. Repeated several times through the day it will keep you wide awake and of more use to your employer.

Knee-Lifts:

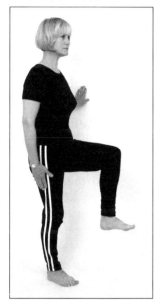

Stand. Hold onto a door handle or whatever to steady you. Slowly raise the right knee until you can feel a stretch in the muscles in the leg. Pull the leg as high as it will go comfortably. Relax and drop the foot to the floor. Raise the left leg and then drop.

Repeat several times on each leg. As you do so you will notice that your knees will lift a tiny bit higher each time. Of course there will be a limit to how high you can lift the knees, but your own body will tell you its own limit. Try to perform at least ten repetitions on each side. Then you will feel a warm glow from the waist down. All the sleepy blood has been turgid in your lower limbs will be circulated back through the system and re-oxygenated.

Windmills:

Stand straight. Swing the right arm in big slow circles such that the inside of your arm swings past the ear as you perform the exercise.

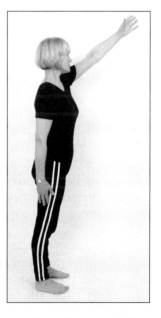

Please remember that windmills turn slowly and thus so should your arms. Swinging the arms quickly I often describe as a propeller. This is not what I want you to do. Take it slowly. Give the muscles in your chest, shoulder and arms time to move and change position without forcing. Muscle doesn't like to have to respond quickly. Complete the exercise by gently swinging the arm forward for ten rotations and then back for ten on the right arm. Then repeat the exercise, both forward and back, on the left arm.

As you swing forward, imagine that you are throwing a cricket ball. As you swing in reverse, imagine that you are in the water in the swimming-pool and that you are reaching for the water behind you. When you have completed this exercise you should feel the same stimulation in the top half of the body as you have done on the bottom with the knee-lifts, and all in all you should now be wide awake and ready for the next bit of the day.

As with anything in life it is sometimes better to stop and think about exercise. Some of the people I know are as lazy as the proverbial 'couch potato'. Simply stated they are happy to lie on the sofa watching television and munching anything that comes to hand. The consequential weight gain and risk to their backs, never mind their general health is of no consequence to them. On the other hand I can think of some zealots who are quite frankly a pain in the butt! They are exercise freaks. At it all the time!

In adults, exercise is important for cardiovascular health, joint function, general physical and mental well being and many other things. The heart is a muscle and needs exercise to keep it in condition. However I am a great advocate of 'everything in moderation'. Thus my final words with regard to exercise are that we all need to do it regularly. However, don't push yourself to the limit. Gradually build to a level that suits you. But keep at it. It will take most folk about three weeks to get to any kind of fit state. If you stop for three weeks the muscles will return to their former condition and you will have to start all of the hard work all over again. So the simple answer is keep at it. Make it a part of your life, for the rest of your life.

However, before we finish with this chapter, allowing that many of the exercises are done on top of a bed, and accepting that when I had severe back pain, simply getting out of bed was a problem, I had no idea how to do it in a manner that was safe. Most of the time, I would twist in the wrong direction and knock my muscles into yet another painful spasm. At times, the simple act of trying to get out of bed caused me major grief. Thus I have developed the following routine that I suggest for anyone suffering with back pain. As with anything that I teach, I hope that you will accept the routine as being sensible, and in doing so will make it your routine for the rest of your life. Getting into bed, is simply the reverse of this routine.

(1) Assuming that you get out of the right side of the bed, then, raise the left leg, to the position shown.

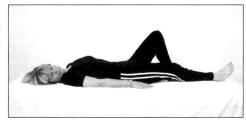

(2) Using the quadriceps muscles (thigh muscles) in the left leg use them to push you onto your right side. At the same time, swing the left arm over and place the hand flat on the bed as shown.

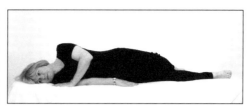

(3) Allow the right leg to fall out of the bed, and the left leg to fall on top of it. In this position you will have created a counter-balance with some of your body weight below the horizontal.

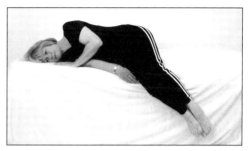

(4) Push with the left hand, while assisting with the right gradually push the body into a vertical position. The legs at the same time will fall towards the floor.

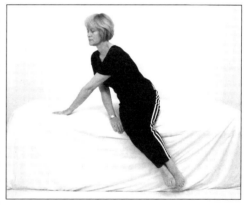

(5) Now place both feet on the floor and with hands by the side, look up (slightly above the horizontal), push with the muscles in the legsand stand up.

There are three receptors in each foot that set up the balance mechanism in the body. Thus it is important that both feet are placed on the floor at the same time.

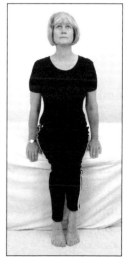

Looking up straightens the thoracic spine (top third of the spine). This in turn helps to straighten the whole of the spine, which in turn helps you to push to an erect position in a pain-free manner.

I ask my patients to make this motto ('look up and stand up') something that they will take with them for the remainder of their lives.

Chapter Nineteen

THE IMPORTANCE OF 'WARM UPS' FOR SPORT

I was fortunate to be asked to work with the physiotherapist at another of Scotland's leading football clubs. He was curious about the therapy I practice and the fact that apparently I was able to resolve physical problems that he couldn't. We struck up a happy relationship and I became used to spending my time working at his club. I had an interest in the complexities of sports injuries. Perhaps more to the point I was keen to prove to him just how good the modality I practice could be in helping to heal these problems quickly.

A week or two into the work and I was approached by a player who told me that had 'hurt himself in the warm-up'. Hurt in the warm up! I could not believe it, yet it seems that such occurrences happen more often than they should at Scottish football clubs. I had the idea that a warm up routine was supposed to be a set of simple exercises designed to gently encourage maximum stretch of the muscles. Then suitably warmed, they should be able to do the work at pace.

Apparently what had happened was that the player had short-circuited the routine. Thus badly prepared, he ran out of the warm dressing room into the cold evening air of the football stadium. When he reached the edge of the pitch, full of exuberance, he held the ball in front and kicked it. It was only then that he realised that he had not stretched off his hamstring muscles. The sudden and violent extension of the muscle tore some of the fibres. The muscle body in response went into painful spasm. Thus the player came limping to looking me for help.

When I had time to think about what he had done I asked him if he had completed any kind of simple pre-warm up in the dressing room. I also asked if he had drunk any water. He told me that he had done neither.

I proceeded to offer the treatment necessary to repair the damaged tissue but as I worked I thought through a simple warm up routine to be executed in the dressing room. I would insist that the players would all have to go through the routine as they changed into their kit. This of course would precede the warm up on the playing field. I discussed it with the club's physiotherapist and we agreed that it was a good idea and that we would adopt it as the regime for all of the players before any training session or club match. We also insisted that all of the players would drink a pint of water while they went through the simple routine that I had devised.

The very next day we had a club match. Every player was given a bottle of water that didn't have a top. The manager explained to the players that from that day they would have to go through this pre-warm up in the dressing room and at the same time drink the pint of water that they had been given. As many of them for whatever reason were against water-drinking the bottles didn't have a top. When all of the players had gone through the routine and were ready to trot off to the warm-up on the pitch, they were all asked to turn the bottles upside down. The simple act of removing the lids allowed that there could be no cheating.

Of course there were howls from the players about the water drinking and in consequence the number of times they would be visiting the toilet. I locked the door of the toilet and put the key in my pocket. When the players returned from the warm-up not one had the need to go the toilet. Their bodies exuded the water through the sweat glands in their skin as they exercised. In very hot surroundings the sweat glands may pour out as much as 10 litres (2 gallons) in a day, together of course with 30 grammes (1oz) of salt. I don't think that the players fully appreciated just how important it is to drink water prior to exercising. Of course Scotland is not a hot country and thus the sweat loss will not be as it would in a hot climate. All the same, in a cold winter's evening it would surprise many a player to see just how much water is lost when playing a fast game of football.

I will write fully about the water drinking in chapter 21. However, for the meantime simply accept the fact that it is very necessary not just to sportsmen and women, but to all of us.

An essential aspect of any sport is fitness preparation. Development of cardio-respiratory fitness, agility, stamina and strength requires an understanding of the subject. Good preparation means fewer injuries. This though depends on a number of factors:

Ventilatory capacity: the amount of air that you can breathe.

Cardiac output: The heart must be able to pump more blood, in response to demand from the exercising muscles. The heart acts as a pump and remains efficient up to about a rate of 180 beats per minute. Above this rate (as when exercising at the maximum) it becomes less efficient as it takes time to fill between each beat. The heart responds to increased demands of exercise by increasing its output of blood. This increased output occurs largely as a result of the increase in rate rather that increase in volume. During exercise the volume pumped with each heart beat increases only slightly.

Blood volume: The circulation becomes less efficient (and therefore oxygen transport less efficient) if large amounts of fluid are lost from the body. During exercise the amount of blood flowing through a muscle increases at least ten-fold. This is achieved partly by widening the vessels, partly by raising the pressure, and partly by opening up new channels. If these new channels are in regular use, they are always available for emergencies (running to catch a bus and such) but if the muscles especially the heart, have not worked for years, then the arteries begin to degenerate and there is nothing in reserve.

Oxygen capacity of the blood: The number and quality of red blood cells should be adequate. Anaemia literally means the lack of blood, but in fact is the shortage haemoglobin, the oxygen carrying pigment of the red blood cells.

Oxygen transport: A most important aspect of fitness to perform strenuous exercise is the individual's ability to transport oxygen to the working muscles. In turn we require the ability to transport oxygen molecules from the air we breathe to the tissues where it is used to create energy.

The lungs: The major function of the lungs concerns the efficient exchange of oxygen and carbon dioxide. Oxygen is necessary in the production of energy and requirements increase dramatically with increasing physical exercise. Carbon dioxide is the end product of many metabolic processes. Hundreds of litres of carbon dioxide must be excreted through the lungs every day.

Distribution of blood to tissues: All parts of the body require an adequate supply of blood in order to function efficiently. However the demands made by the different parts are neither equal nor constant. When your body is at rest the 'vegetative' functions such as digestion and production of urine are promoted. Much of the blood is diverted to the small intestine (to absorb the end products of digestion) and the kidneys (to be purified). When the body undergoes strenuous physical activity, much blood is diverted to the skeletal activities where it is required to provide additional supplies of oxygen and glucose for energy release.

I have described a warm-up routine in chapter 9 that I find suitable for golfers. This warm-up can be used though for any sport. Additionally if you are a sporty type after completing the warm-up as described (except for the bit with the golf club) a jog around the perimeter of a sports ground is good.

You should be clad in a warm tracksuit and you should jog in a relaxed way, to allow the muscles, heart and lungs to function in their most physiological manner in preparation for the heavy stress that you will apply later when exercising at full pelt.

For those of us with back pain though the answer is to keep it simple. The golf warm up or even the knee-lifts and windmills will suffice before heading out for a good long walk. I think that few people would deny that exercise promotes good health. Exercise strengthens muscles and disuse causes them to waste. For a back pain sufferer once some sort of normality has been reached and your pain level has diminished and your mobility improved it would be my opinion that exercise is of the utmost importance. Health cannot be measured as muscular strength. Exercise thus has more subtle effects. As far as I understand for people with high blood pressure the mortality rate is highest in those who don't take any exercise. Of course this is influenced by over eating, smoking, which are contributory factors.

Vigorous exercise results in reflective changes occurring in the body's internal environment. The metabolic (the chemical changes by which foods are converted into components of the body or consumed as fuel) rate rise in skeletal muscles that are hard at work.

However, before we get too deep in trying to understand the complexities of a human being, I am sure that you will agree that exercise is important to our survival. I like living and being alive. I don't know what is going to happen after I die. No one does. Thus I take my exercise and the health that it gives me very seriously. I am not at the gym at 6.00 every morning such as some people I can think of but I do exercise frequently in the form of regular games of golf in the summer and good longs walks in the winter months where, despite the persistent wet weather that we experience in the west of Scotland. I enjoy getting wrapped up and out in the fresh air.

Additionally I appreciate that when I exercise and keep fit (even to a reasonable level) it keeps my back muscles in good order and less likely to be hurt. I always go though my warm-up routine no matter what form my exercise is going to take. As far as I am concerned it is just too important.

Chapter Twenty

GOOD EATING and HEALTHY FOODS

Daoists say: "What you put into your body is what you get out of it!"

How many times have you been standing at the checkout at the supermarket and find yourself staring into the trolley of the shopper next to you? I do it all the time. Call me nosey if you wish but I cannot stop myself. Of course there is a feeling of self-importance in this. My subconscious implies a facial expression probably with a self-righteous smirk that if you could read it would say, "The contents of my trolley are better than yours". Of course I am foolish to adopt such a stance even if I don't actually speak any words. However allowing for the wholesome and healthy regime that I use to sustain my body I may have some justification. As you are aware I live in Scotland and thus will only speak about the diet in this country. There must a semblance of analogy in other parts of the world.

As far as I am concerned we simply don't eat the right type of food. We are fatter than we should be. Our children are worse. Obesity is on the increase and in my opinion must be a contributory factor leading to back pain in later life. The children of today don't play in the streets as we did. How many of them have the summer jobs that I had as an energetic youngster? The picture I painted about my lifestyle and all of the work that I have done throughout indicated that perhaps my spare time jobs such as picking potatoes and the like could have added to my back problem. The point is though that despite my back pain that at least I got off my backside and went looking for a job. I have worked and been busy all of my life. In today's world it seems that many children spend their time in front of a TV screen or a Playstation? Additionally how many of them, indeed how many of us, have the five portions of green vegetables or fruit on a daily basis that our bodies need to survive?

Thus, in Scotland as we queue at the check-out in the supermarket, I shudder when I look into the trolleys of other people who have been shopping. Why, oh why, do they insist in purchasing tinned potatoes and vegetables when fresh ones are so cheap and easy to cook? Why is the fresh fish rejected in favour of the frozen variety wrapped in batter? Why do we purchase so many 'ready meals' produced in factories that include in the packet all sorts of chemicals and preservatives, mostly surreptitiously? Is it just that we are now a lazy nation wishing to spend all of our free time before the television? Have we become a nation of watchers rather than participators? Football in Scotland comes before anything. In this country we are amongst the best spectators in the world. At the recent football world cup held in Germany the Scotland football team failed to qualify. Yet despite a team to support there was a Scotland flag prominent at every single match played. But at what cost to our health? Scots (at least some of us) really do eat those soggy grey 'Scotch' pies, with the fillings resembling the mangled remains from the inside of somebody's brain? I have to admit that in the dim and distant past I have succumbed and consumed such an uncongenial and downright unhealthy item. Thus what an unhealthy story our shopping trolleys tell.

In my opinion the adults are to blame. We have forgotten the youthful vigour of the street games we played. We have allowed our children to become slovenly. How many times in the morning have you been walking down a street behind some children shuffling to school and breakfasting on bags of crisps and fizzy drinks? There is no great surprise to read of an obesity time bomb among our young – with children under four showing signs of being tubby and one in ten diagnosed as obese. This of course raises all sorts of serious health problems in the future, not to say the problems that they may have with back pain in their adult lives. The Government protests that they are doing all they can. In reality they are doing nothing.

Although there is very little evidence of the diet of prehistoric man, I understand that archaeologists have discovered tools and food residues that give us some idea as to their eating habits. Our ancestors relied on hunting and fishing for their food supplies. They ate what they could catch or what they could find that was growing wild. They had to expend a great deal of energy in this process. The food was eaten raw.

Eventually man discovered fire that meant that his food could now be roasted or boiled. If you think about the difference between raw and cooked potato then you can imagine just how important this discovery was. In time we learned to farm. Cultivation replaced seed gathering. Wild animals were domesticated. Agricultural methods slowly evolved. However man had no mechanical implements to help. He was totally reliant on manual labour. Apart from salting or drying he had no means of food preserving. People had to use local produce for the majority of their food.

Detailed records of life in medieval times in the UK show that the basic staple foods remained unchanged for thousands of years. Most meals were based on vegetables. Bread was made from locally ground rye and wheat flours. Fresh meat and fish were eaten in the summer, but had to be salted for the winter. Honey was the most common sweetener. Beer was the most common drink.

The change from that somewhat basic diet to what we have in the modern world progressed very slowly at first. Voyagers to the new world brought back unusual foods such as potato, tea and coffee. Sugar, which was initially grown only from sugar cane, was imported only as an expensive luxury. It did not become a household commodity until 200 years ago. Our choice of food began to expand. However, it was the industrial revolution that had the greatest impact with the advances in transport. Thus in the last hundred years the need to grow food locally has disappeared.

In the last thirty years or so refrigeration has come to the fore. Consequently we now have access to foods from all over the world. Then again, how much of this is good for us?

The way we purchase food is changing rapidly. Much of what we eat today has been chemically processed in one way or another. Raw materials are rarely sold as grown but are processed. How many of us cook a pot of soup? We would all rather purchase something in a tin. This is despite the fact that it is probably full of monosodium glutamate and other horrible chemicals. These changes in food availability began about a hundred years ago. During the war years we had austerity and food shortages. However since then things have accelerated.

We enjoy twentieth century food but we still have the body of prehistoric man. How much of this food we need depends on our total activity. Our ancestors spent most of their time chasing after the food they were trying to eat. We have it presented on a plate. We have thus two problems. We eat more than we need and in the course of eating most of what we devour is rubbish. We are harming our bodies piling on the calories, which in turn become fat layers under the skin. We put on additional weight. The spine has to take the strain. Too much strain leads to back problems.

Food today is advertised and packaged in an appealing way. It is quick to digest and contains lots of salt and sugar, which in turn blunts our appetite mechanism and leads to many of us becoming overweight. There is a decreased fibre content in the food. The mix of foods we eat no longer matches our requirements and as a result I can see that there has been an increase in ill health. It would seem to me that this is directly related to our eating habits.

We have often heard it said that Mediterranean people live longer healthier lives. It is suggested that the secret is in the food they eat. It would be impossible for us to follow the diet but there are many patterns in the diet we can broadly follow. Their fat intake consists of olive oil more than any other fat. More fish than meat is consumed, as are moderate amounts of wine. Activity plays a vital part. The people of the Mediterranean incorporate exercise into their daily lives.

Exercise is vital for good health and the best weight. So in accepting that prevention is better than cure we are agreeing with the Mediterranean philosophy. Their diet contains protective substances, essential fatty acids, high amounts of fibre and anti oxidants, fish, fresh fruit and vegetables, and of course olive oil. Olive oil is the healthier choice at the supermarket because it is low in saturated fat and high in mono-unsaturated fat.

Fish oil has always been high on my agenda. In my opinion fish are medicine. Few foods have more curative and healing properties than oil-rich fish. Tinned tuna seems to be the exception in that most of the polyunsaturated omega-3 fats are lost in the cooking process. However wild Pacific salmon, sardines, mackerel, pilchards and anchovies are real super-foods! In addition scientists have suggested that people who eat this sort of diet have higher levels of the "feel good" hormone serotonin and are less likely to suffer from depression. Eskimos suffer less from coronary heart disease as the oils interfere with blood-clotting mechanisms. The latest studies have revealed that fish oils might be a useful tool in repairing cartilage breakdown in knee joints. Perhaps the same repair is taking place in the ligaments in the spine?

Anyone who suffers with back pain back must have a sensible diet and at least take some regular exercise. These two principles must go hand in hand. Thus I try to eat sensibly. I follow the Mediterranean example. I am working hard at reducing my weight. I exercise five times a week. Not being one for the gymnasium I am happy to plug in the headphones in my little portable radio and head off at a good pace down the adjacent country lanes. In the dark winter nights I am just as happy to drive into town, park the car and take a route around the shops. I also eat virtually no salt, much less sugar and fat and more fibre. I am by no means the perfect specimen. However in recent years I have tried to become a better person. Walking has become something that I enjoy. It is no longer a chore. If you are a back pain sufferer then perhaps you will follow the same example.

Over the years I have published a number of newsletters from my clinic in Glasgow. In this I would include a variety of news, health tips and indeed anything that would help my patients. As part if this and allowing for the fact that I was in 1999 a finalist in the BBC Radio Scotland Personality Super-Cook competition I have always included a healthy recipe or two.

I am one of these sorts of fellows who live to eat rather than eat to live. However I accept that what you eat is a powerful key to health. In turn if I eat too much I will get fat. If I get fat my muscles will struggle to cope carrying the extra weight of my big fat belly. Then my back pain will return. My body wants to be well but often my eating habits have created problems that could have been avoided. This is because some of the substances in food are changed by the body's chemistry into other substances which have undesirable effects. In essence our bodies are little chemical factories.

Fat is one of those substances. It can be transformed into excess cholesterol. Too much cholesterol in the blood can lead to narrowing of the arteries and add to the risk of heart disease. The amount of cholesterol that we produce depends on several factors but the type of fat that you eat is a major factor. Cholesterol levels vary from one person to another and combined with tobacco smoking and raised blood pressure make up three major risk factors for heart disease. A simple test at your doctor or pharmacist will reveal your cholesterol level. We all produce cholesterol naturally in our bodies. A white waxy substance, it is an essential component of cell membranes of most tissues. It is also found in foods of animal origin such as meat, milk, butter, cheese, cream and eggs.

Saturated fat is something that I get very angry about. It is added to all sorts of foods with the worst culprits being cakes, chocolates, biscuits, crisps, and ice-cream and meat pies. Vegetable sources of saturated fat are coconut oil and palm oil. Producers use them all the time, so my advice is that when you shop, and you do have some sort of processed food or another – read the label. If you don't and end up consuming saturated fat in large quantities you will find that your body will use the fat to make cholesterol.

Polyunsaturated fats are found mostly in vegetable foods and polyunsaturated vegetable oils such as sunflower, maize or corn. They cannot be eaten with abandon but can largely replace saturated fats.

Mono-unsaturated fats are found in foods such as avocados, olives, peanuts and olive oil and peanut oil. They do not raise your cholesterol level but are high in kilojoules and should be limited.

When people ask me if I have a recipe for a healthy life I respond by telling them that they should enjoy everything in moderation.

Eat a wide variety of foods. Keep a healthy weight check. Eat fewer fatty foods. Don't smoke. Drink lots of water. Exercise as often as you can and daily if at all possible. Drink less alcohol. Cut out the salt intake. We will find salt in bread that forms a daily part of many lives. It is thus not necessary to add any when cooking. I don't! Eat more roughage – porridge, wholemeal bread, vegetables and fruit. The skin on the fruit is valuable roughage. However I accept that more than likely it has been sprayed with some sort of chemical or other, thus when I bring fruit home with me, the first thing that I do is wash it in soap and water and rinse with clean water before putting it in the fruit bowl.

Talking about fruit, an Italian lady who was once a patient at my clinic told me that in Italy people purchase their fruit on a daily basis and consume it more or less as soon as they get home. Here in Scotland most of the folk that I know take the fruit home and place it into their fruit-bowl where it may remain for a week or more. Fruit, according to my Italian friend, is meant to eaten on the day of purchase. The lady was a good cook. She was, as I am, interested in food. Thus, as I would treat her, we would often talk about one type of cooking or another. In the course of this she gave me a recipe for tomato soup that I will, with her permission, share with you. Of course this is a book about back pain and not a cookery book. However I don't think that it will matter to give you a few of the better recipes that I have found in different parts of the world.

Tomato Soup

Ingredients:

2 large potatoes
3 carrots
3 shallots
1 tablespoon of olive oil
1 kg of good quality ripe tomatoes, washed,
or two tins of Italian plum tomatoes
1.5 litres of ham stock (see note # as under)
Black pepper

Method:

Clean and peel the potatoes carrots and shallots. Then if you have food processor shred them coarsely. If not take the time to grate all of the vegetables.

Add the oil to a saucepan. Then add the shredded vegetables and cook over a low heat for about 30 minutes turning often. Keep the lid on the saucepan and don't let the vegetables burn. If you have to, add a tablespoon of cold water from time to time. Then add the tomatoes, stalks skins and all. Mix all of the ingredients together and allow cooking for a further 15 minutes or so until the tomatoes have softened down. Sometimes in the winter when the quality of tomatoes is not so good I will add a tin of Italian plum tomatoes to the fresh ones. The combination works just as well.

After this combination is cooked through, place the mixture a little at a time into a conical sieve. I bought one some years ago and find it invaluable. Use a wooden spoon to push the mixture through the holes in the sieve and allow the juice to fall into a bowl. Dump the debris from the mixture left in the sieve onto your compost heap if you have one, or at least dispose of it organically if you can. (The same applies to the tins that contained the tomatoes). Then it is time to add the ham stock.

(Note #)

There are a number of alternatives with regard to ham stock. (a) If you have an organic butcher near you (one that you can trust) I would purchase a ham knuckle (known in Scotland as a ham-end). (b) If not and you have to purchase a piece of ham from a supermarket where Lord knows what sort of process it has gone through I would firstly wash it. Then I would soak it covered in a big pan of cold water for 24 hours, changing the water twice. In this way it may be possible to get some of the chemicals out of it. I suppose that I should say that I rarely purchase smoked ham as I don't know what or how it has been cured.

On the few occasions that I have used such a piece of meat I bring it to the boil. Pour off the water and then refill with cold water. Then I will simmer the meat with just a large potato in the pan with it. The potato should help to remove any residual salt from the water. I would remove the meat to cool and dispose of the potato. Then I would reduce the stock to the volume required for the soup. (c) The third option is to purchase a stock cube. There are lots of varieties to choose from. However if you examine the label you should be able to find one with the least amount of salt. I am able to source some in a good organic health food shop in Glasgow. I will leave this to your own common sense.

Add the ham stock to the sieved potato, tomato mix and bring to the boil. Simmer for a few minutes and just before the finish add some fresh black pepper. I often make this soup and take it with me to the clinic. I don't like to eat when working; I probably often miss lunch due to the clinic hours I work. However I am happy to sip from my own hot home-made soup. Alternatively if serving at home, add a scatter of freshly chopped parsley or torn basil leaves (if in season). The cold boiled ham, if you have it, will be great for sandwiches.

I am sorry to say this but as you may have guessed I am a lover of Italian and French food and cooking methods. A book (Cuisine Minceur) written in 1977 by Michel Guérard, a chef of some repute was a great inspiration. I don't have his permission to reproduce any of his recipes but I can let you know that in the introduction to the book he wrote that he awoke one morning with the weight of his belly holding him on the bed. His life as a chef increased the number of centimetres that it took to measure the girth of his waist. He goes on to say that he had further reason to lose some pounds (kilos) to gain the hand in marriage of the woman he loved. Thus he produced this innovative cookery book that contains so many excellent recipes. In a way he lets us into the secret of how to cook yet not to use the cream, butter and rich delectable sauces that are so much a part of French cooking.

However, for the sake of providing yet another good recipe and to take you now to a main course I return to a friend who, as with my father, was an engineer on a ship. His journeys took him mostly round the Mediterranean ports. In such a port he gleaned the following recipe while dining one evening at a small local restaurant. The recipe is apparently well known and often used in Italy yet I find it rarely used in restaurants here. Allowing that it has such a fantastic flavour I don't know why. The dish is known as spaghetti putanesca and originated in Naples where it was named after local women of easy virtue.

Spaghetti Putanesca

Ingredients: (serves four)

4 tbsp of olive oil (I always try to buy the
best quality first pressing)
2 cloves of garlic finely chopped
¼ teaspoon of chilli powder
1 x 2 oz can of anchovy fillets chopped
12 oz tomatoes, fresh, skinned, de-seeded
and chopped

2 tbsp of capers, rinsed and chopped
1 cup of back stoned olives, halved
1 tbsp of tomato paste
1 lb of spaghetti
2 tbsp of fresh chopped parsley to serve

Method:

Bring a large pan of water to the boil

While this is heating add the oil to a frying pan. I have a cast-iron skillet that I purchased years ago that has and will last for years, which I find excellent for cooking such dishes as it spreads the heat from my gas stove so well.

Add the garlic and chilli to the oil and cook for 2-3 minutes until the garlic is golden but not burned. Add the anchovies and mash them into the garlic with a fork. Add the tomatoes, capers and tomato paste and stir well. Put a lid on the pan and allow cooking over a medium heat.

Now add the spaghetti to the now boiling water. Stir and cook until it is just *al dente.* Drain.

Turn the spaghetti into the sauce and fold all the ingredients together. Raise the heat and cook for a few minutes, then serve with a sprinkling of fresh chopped parsley. Don't allow anyone to sprinkle with cheese. It just doesn't go with this recipe.

Having given you a recipe for a starter soup and a main course I thought that it would now be time for a pudding. As a boy I loved my mother's rice pudding. Made with full-fat milk it was a joy as my brother and my two sisters fought over the burned skin that would form on the surface as it baked in the oven. It makes me wonder why we did this. I suppose is a bit like drinking the froth of the top of my dad's beer.

In actual fact the sour taste of the beer was awful. Yet, I strived to convince dad that he should allow me to scoop up the foaming froth that quickly filled my mouth and more often than not made me choke with the humongous amount of gas bubbles that it contained.

I just love fruit. It is natural, God given, fulfilling and just downright yummy to eat when it is in season. Speaking about seasons, I played some golf at my local course recently. We are fortunate to have two courses: one of 18 holes (that is sometimes used as the qualifying course when the Open comes to Troon) and another of nine holes. My partners and I would normally play on the bigger course. However last evening it was a dull drizzly Scottish summer evening and thus we decided to play over the shorter course. It had been some weeks, months since we played this course.

Arriving at the third tee I was surprised to see a host of wild raspberry bushes loaded with fruit. I happily scoffed on a handful or two while my golf partners looked on in amazement. "Covered in bird shit" was all they could say. There was no way that they would consider eating such wild fruit. Yet, this takes me back to the caveman. Our ancestors! They ate the fruit in the wild much as I did on the golf course. I ate raspberry contaminated with exhaust fumes from aircraft engine fuel and all of the other pollutants that we have to deal with these days. On the other hand our ancestors had to eat the same fruit polluted with volcanic ash, pterodactyl droppings or whatever. In essence despite a difference of a million years or so nothing has changed.

So, as a fruit lover who accepts the benefits I now offer my vision of wonderfulness, a dish that gives me the hope that I am preserving my health by giving my body the fuel to help it fight disease. Eating should evoke a sense of delight, excitement and interest.

Hippocrates' famous statement about 'food is medicine' is inspiring just as long as everything to do with it doesn't feel or taste like medicine. I want to feel invigorated after a meal. In the dark days of my past I would eat a pizza and follow it with a tub of ice-cream. After such a meal I would be lethargic, lie on the sofa and forego the after-dinner walk in the park. In all I was a pig. Today I am a different person. I have enjoyed a supper of herring toasted in oatmeal, pan fried in just a little olive oil and served with steamed carrots, peas and sweet corn. Half an hour later and I am writing up the words of this chapter full of energy gained from my delicious repast.

Fruit platter with redcurrant sauce

Ingredients: (to serve about ten folk if you are having a dinner party. Adjust the proportion if not – or save the remainder in the fridge for tomorrow).

2 mangoes

They don't grow mangoes in Scotland and thus I have to accept with dignity that in allowing an airline to fly this product from the other side of the world I am in a way doing my bit to harm the environment. On the other hand if the mango came to the UK in a temperature controlled ship then I don't feel so bad. Mango is such a wonderful fruit that I find myself like a wee boy stealing a bit of chocolate when I eat it. Anyway allowing that it is a treat that happens just once in a while I hope hat you will allow the mango vice. It is of course assumed that all of the fruit is ripe and ready to eat.

2 x 250g punnets of strawberries
½ a melon, sliced
2 pears sliced
2 apples sliced
2 bananas sliced
6 kiwi fruit sliced
½ a cup of passion fruit pulp (from about six passion fruit)

Arrange the fruit in alternate varieties in a clockwise direction or (anti-clockwise if it suits) on a big bright platter

Ingredients for the redcurrant sauce
200g of frozen or fresh redcurrants
2 tbsp of Manuka honey (New Zealand)
1 tbsp of water
1 tbsp of cornflour

2 tbsp of Grand Marnier (well, we all need a wee bit of alcohol now and again. Between ten folk it's not going to any harm. It does though add to the flavour).

Combine the redcurrants, water and honey in a pan. Bring to the boil and simmer, covered for a few minutes. Allow to cool slightly and blend in a processor. I try to do this with short sharp blasts in the blender such that the fruit pulp in the redcurrants is broken to pieces but not the redcurrant seeds. Push the pulp through a fine sieve. Return the mixture to the pan. Blend the cornflour with a little water and heat though until the sauce thickens a little. Allow to cool and stir in the liqueur.

Serve the jug of sauce with the fruit platter and let your guests enjoy the vivid array of colours and the succulent fruit.

With supper over, a while later it will be time for bed. I often have some mint tea a simple yet delicious night-time treat. I am lucky to have a mint bush in the garden. It grows in a big pot that I buried in the ground some years ago. Encapsulated like this it will continue to grow happily for many years to come. The problem with mint is that if you plant it in the ground it will spread and take over a corner of any well tended garden.

And so to my tea: pull a few young stalks from the top of a shoot and place in the bottom of a cup. Boil some water and pour over the leaves. Leave for a few minutes to brew. Sip and enjoy.

When I was first introduced to this drink I would spit the leaves out as they came to my lips. Now I am happy to chew the goodness of the leaves as they float to the surface as I drink this refreshing draft. Then I am off to bed for a good night's sleep.

I cannot leave this chapter without finishing with a story about breakfast food. During the week I will alternate my breakfast between a good plate of porridge and a smoothie. The porridge I make with water. I always give it a good whisk as it cooks. After cooking for a few minutes I will stir in a tablespoon of Manuka or other best quality honey and a little skimmed milk. Alternatively I will add half a grated apple and a pinch of cinnamon.

The smoothie I probably take on days when I am busy and don't have a lot of time before leaving for the clinic. I have a couple of recipes to offer:

Half of a sliced mango
A banana
A handful of fresh raspberries or strawberries
(or frozen berries)
Freshly squeezed orange juice
Dump the ingredients into a blender and
zizz for a minute or so.

This smoothie has a bit of bulk and is very satisfying. Quite frankly it is my crutch when I am in a hurry to get to the clinic. Many a busy day has been 'smoothed' by regular sips from this wholesome luxury drink as I work.

I should at this point advise that I am against modern smoothie making machines. They will force the juice from anything that you place in them. The problem that I have with them is that they also remove all of the pith and pulp that is important as roughage in our digestion. My old-fashioned blender doesn't do this.

Another zingy smoothie that I enjoy again doesn't have a name. However here are the ingredients. It is quite yummy. I find it refreshing on a Saturday morning when I don't have work to go to but have the time to sit and enjoy it as I read the morning paper.

1 litre of apple juice
A small piece of root ginger peeled and chopped
3 kiwi fruits peeled and roughly chopped
3 satsumas peeled
1 pineapple peeled cored and roughly chopped
Juice of one lime

Put the apple juice and the ginger in a blender and liquidise for a few seconds. The ginger is quite a tough stringy material but adds a brilliant and succinct touch to the flavour. Thus it is best to whizz until it has been macerated. Then pour the mix through a sieve to remove any pith. Pour the liquid back into the blender. Add the other ingredients and blend. In the summer I serve this with some chunks of ice when it is a wonderful cooler on a hot day. I think that the ginger has something to do with the cooling, but perhaps it is a bit of nonsense that I picked up on one of my travels.

Finally, I suppose that I cannot finish a chapter such as this without having a word about the 'bad guys': companies who produce large volumes of 'so-called' healthy drinks. Invariably they are supported with massive advertising campaigns often targeted at children. These products are billed as containing real fruit. In reality they contain massive amounts of sugar – as much as seven teaspoonfuls per can. It would be my opinion that this will lead the children to have a sweet tooth in years to come and affect the eating habits in years to come. Sugary drinks can cause tooth decay and weight gain and eventually back pain caused by all of the extra weight that the people who drink them will eventually have to lump around. If you have any sense, steer clear of such deceitfully advertised products. Real fruit with skin on that you have to peel yourself is the only answer.

But enough! I will get off my high-horse. Good eating and healthy foods just have to be part of life. I hope that you agree that there are many ingredients in weight control. However, if you give your body a chance by reducing some of your excess poundage, you will in turn be helping your back pain problems.

Chapter Twenty One

THE IMPORTANCE OF DRINKING WATER

The human body was developed from a species that were given life in water, which allowed that the dependence on the life giving properties was inherited. Thus we all know that we need water to survive. Every cell, tissue, organ and body process requires water. We need the water to carry food, minerals and vitamins via the blood stream to the various parts of our bodies. Water transports away toxins and it also helps to regulate our body temperature. We could last up to 10 weeks without food, but we would die after 10 days without water. The human body is composed of 25% solid matter and 75% water. The brain is said to consist of 85% water. In death the energetic framework collapses and we dry out. We return to dust. In life it is the solvent – the water content – that regulates all functions of the body.

My understanding is that we should drink three pints (1.5 litres) of water every day. There is no need to purchase expensive mineral water, but you can if you wish and you have the money for it. The French are mad about it. In the morning I fill a jug, place a piece of kitchen paper on top to keep out the dust and simply leave it sitting on the kitchen table for an hour or so. The water from the tap will probably contain fluoride and chlorine (a bacteria killing agent) to keep it in pristine condition as it passes through the pipes. Leaving it for a while allows the chemicals to evaporate, with the result that the water then tastes just as it should when it left the loch, lake or reservoir from whence it came. As the day goes on, each time I pass the jug I will have a sip; a mouthful at a time. Thus during the day and with little effort I am able to drink my three pints. I have water all over the place: in bottles in the car, at my desk in the office, beside my bed! I have it everywhere.

Thus I am continually sipping the water as the day goes by. I probably don't drink too much in the hours before going to bed, as it would keep me awake by having to visit the bathroom. Most of my water drinking is during the day. My body has become used to it.

If you agree and start to drink water on a regular basis, you may find that your bladder, at first, will find it difficult to cope and you will probably run to the toilet a bit more than you should do. The bladder is a muscular sac that distends as fluid is (temporarily) stored and whose contraction ejects the fluid at the appropriate time. The dimensions of the urinary bladder vary with its state of distension, but a full urinary bladder can contain as much as a litre of urine. Gradually as you get into the water-drinking routine it will come to terms with having to hold onto a bit more water than it used to do. Your liver and kidneys will love you for the extra fluid, helping to flush out all the toxins. By drinking water we can re-hydrate the skin, maximise the immune system, increase concentration, help prevent constipation and lower the risk of developing gallstones and kidney stones. Water is very much part of our very existence. We need to keep our bodies well supplied with it. With only a very small decrease in your body's normal water content you quickly feel thirsty. 1% or 2% deficiency can be distressing and painful. 5% deficiency can cause skin shrinkage, dried out mouth and tongue, and hallucinations can begin. A 15% loss usually results in death.

From a back pain point of view water is the important lubricant that keeps the muscle tissues in a fluid state. Muscle is the most abundant tissue in the body. It consists of two fifths of body weight. It is made of muscle fibre, a long slender cell or agglomeration of cells that become shorter and thicker in response to stimulus. The fibres are supported and bound together by ordinary connective tissue. There are three types of muscle. Cardiac, is the substance of the heart. Smooth, is found in the walls of the digestive and urinary tracts.

Striated, is our flesh - lean meat. From a back pain point of view striated muscle is of importance. It is composed of bands of fibres each about 1/1000mm wide. The fibres must have a lubricant to allow them to slide past each other, much as a car engine has oil as the lubricant, our bodies need plain water as the lubricant for the muscle fibres.

A muscle's design is similar to an orange where a thick skin (fascia) encases the whole of the fruit. Deeper layers of fascia separate the orange into 'wedges'. A thin coating of tissue surrounds each individual tiny 'bud' of fruit. Applying this analogy to muscle, a layer of fascia encases the muscle belly. A deeper layer wraps the long muscle fibres into bundles. Each microscopic fibre is bound in fascia. Unlike an orange the muscle's connective tissues merge at either end to form a strong tendon. The tendon attaches the muscle to the bone. Muscle tissue is unique because it can be in a relaxed or contracted state. When the muscle is relaxed it has a soft malleable feel. When contracted it has a firm, solid quality. However the reason for telling you all of this is to try to make you understand that muscles can only operate when they are properly hydrated and lubricated with plain water!

By the way, it is my understanding that the body looks at water in different ways. Taking plain water and the body says thank you and sends it straight to where it is needed most. Taking in water with added fruit syrup and the body looks at it as food and directs it through the system in another way.

I wrote about drinking water in relation to the importance of warm ups for sport and my amazement that footballers and other such athletes can 'injure themselves in the warm up'. It is obvious to me that they are simply not taking enough water on board before they start to exercise. This is the reason why I would advocate drinking a pint of water at the same time as completing a pre-warm up routine in the dressing room.

Our bodies are constantly losing water. In addition to the two pints normally lost through the skin and the breath, another three pints or more may be eliminated through our kidneys and bowels. Water is also lost by sweating and even by tears. Thus we need about five or six pints of fluid on a daily basis. The body will find this in many ways. It will take it from dry bread if it has to. Of course this is hard on the system and thus it is obvious to make it easier and give it plain water. Our bodies produce water (about a pint a day) as a by-product as it amalgamates the glucose from the food we eat with the oxygen we breathe to form our energy source, Adenosine Triphosphate (ATP) – that keeps us going throughout the day.

It should be appreciated that the spinal joints, intervertebral joints and their disc structures are dependent on the different hydraulic properties of water. In spinal vertebral joints, water is not only a lubricant for the contact surfaces but is also held in the disc core and supports the compression weight of the upper part of the body. Fully 75% of the weight of the upper part of the body is supported by the water volume that is stored in the disc core. 25% is supported by the fibrous material around the disc. In all joints, water acts as a lubricating agent. It bears the force produced by weight. Joint movement causes a vacuum to be created in the joint space. Water will be pulled through the bone and cartilage into the joint – if it is available. Without water there is no lubrication between the cartilages that wraps the end of all bones. Cartilage rubbing against itself will quickly wear away, leaving the bone to rub against itself. Then we develop arthritic joints.

Whereas bone cells are immersed in calcium deposits, the

cartilage cells are immersed in a matrix containing much water. As the cartilage surfaces glide over one another, some exposed cells die and peel away and new cells take their place.

In a well-hydrated cartilage, the rate of friction damage is minimal, on the other hand, in a de-hydrated cartilage; the rate of frictional damage is increased.

With particular regard to low back pain it should be appreciated that the spinal joints are dependant on different hydraulic properties of water stored in the disc core, as well as the end plate cartilage covering the flat surfaces of the spinal vertebrae. In spinal joints, water is the lubricant between the contact surfaces. We simply just cannot do without it. Even more so if you suffer with back pain of any kind.

In trying to prevent back pain, drinking water should be combined with a series of gentle exercises (as I have explained). These exercises will help create an intermittent vacuum that in turn draws water into the disc space. The exercises in turn will help to reduce the risk of muscle spasm that in the vast majority of people is the main cause of lower back pain. Rheumatoid arthritic joints and their pain are to be viewed as indicators of water deficiency in the affected joint cartilage surfaces.

Statistics show that in the UK as many as 20 million people suffer with joint symptoms, of which four million are disabled by arthritis. A further 20 million in any year will have to endure back pain. Once any of these conditions is established in an individual, it becomes a sentence for suffering for the remainder of the individual's life, unless that is we do something about it.

Water of course has more to do in the body than simply help reduce back pain. To give an example, let me tell you a tale.

A fellow I know (lets call him Willie) told me that he had gone to his doctor for examination. He told the doctor that he was suffering with dizzy spells and altogether he did not feel good. The doctor listened to his story and then asked that he check his blood pressure. The readings were not good. The doctor (who was an old fellow) told Willie that all was not well and that he would have to watch what he was doing. He prescribed some pills and asked Willie to return for another check two weeks later.

Willie went home and told his wife the tale. When out shopping the next day, they came across a shop that sold blood pressure monitors. They decided to make a purchase. Despite the fact that I know that these do-it-yourself machines are lacking in accuracy, they will give some indication as to what is going on. To say the least, over the next week as Willie checked his blood pressure it was as he said "all over the place".

Willie returned to the doctor for another check. Again the doctor told him that his blood pressure was not good and prescribed yet another batch of pills. The dizzy spells continued as did the erratic blood pressure readings. Willie was not a happy fellow at all.

After another few days with this horrible situation he returned once again to his doctor, where he was to find that the old man had gone off on holiday and had been replaced with a new, young, lady doctor, fresh out of college. She carried out the necessary checks and had a look at as his medical history. She then told Willie that she didn't like the concoction of pills that he was consuming on a daily basis. She asked for a blood sample and told Willie that she would send it off to the lab for analysis. She would let him know the results as soon as she had them.

The next day Willie got a phone call from the young doctor. She told him that she had the results from the blood test and advised that the mixture of pills he was consuming were harming his liver. She told him to stop taking them and come to see her immediately. When Willie arrived at the clinic, the doctor did not look happy. She asked Willie all sorts of questions about his health and in the process enquired as to how much fluid (water) he had as a daily intake. Willie told her that he had one or two cups of black coffee. The doctor was aghast. She told him to stop taking all of the pills and immediately to increase his fluid (water) intake to three pints daily. She told him to return for another consultation again two weeks later.

When Willie returned to the clinic at the appointed time, he told the doctor that his dizzy spells had gone. When the doctor checked his blood pressure she found it to be normal. The doctor then explained (as I have) that the blood in the system is 92% water. However, with such a low fluid intake, Willie's blood was like treacle. Every time he stood up the blood could not go with him. Thus there was a shortage of blood getting to the brain and inconsequence, the dizzy spells. Now that he had a proper amount of fluid in his body the blood was able to flow around the system much easier and when he stood the blood flow to the brain was uninterrupted. Of course Willie is now a convert to water drinking.

The colour of urine, by the way should not be dark. It should ideally be colourless to light yellow. If it begins to become dark yellow, or even an orange sort of colour, it is a sign of dehydration. In essence the kidneys will be working hard to get rid of the toxins, which in turn is why urine becomes darker in colour.

I could write a whole book about water drinking. In my life and in that of all of my family it is an important part of our existence. All of the patients who come to me for treatment are given a good physical examination and consequential treatment, while at the same time I work on trying to convince them as I hope I have convinced you of the importance of water drinking. There are many other aspects of human life that are touched by water usage, other than I have described here. In these few words though I hope that you can agree with me and if necessary take one step in your life to make it just that little bit better.

Chapter Twenty Two

CHINESE MEDICINE, ACUPUNCTURE, CHIROPRATIC and OTHERS

In the dark days, when I struggled to come to terms with my doctor telling me to prepare for life in a wheelchair, I knew nothing of alternative medicine. It was a world that simply to me did not exist. All I knew was that I had exhausted the traditional forms of medicine that I knew of at the time.

One day I met a fellow who had similar problems to me. He told me about a chiropractor who had moved to the area. Apparently he was able to sort backs. I was scared at first. Chiropractic was new to Scotland and I knew very little about it. Some sort of body engineering I assumed. There were very few practitioners. However I decided to give it a go and telephoned for an appointment. On the first visit the practitioner took an X-ray. After developing it, it was placed on a screen to illuminate the picture. I was told that I had the spine of an old man, but with a bit of manipulation it could be helped.

I lay on the treatment table not knowing what was to happen. The practitioner pushed a knee into my back, held onto my shoulders and pulled hard. I heard some clicking and crunching noises. Then my upper spine was manipulated, this time by laying me prone with my face through a hole in the table and pressing hard with his hands. Again I could hear some sort of clicking noises. Finally he turned me onto my back and stood at my head. Holding it with both hands he snapped it from one side to another, and all in an instant. I was shocked. However I arose from the treatment table and on the whole I was pain free. In addition I seemed to be standing straight. A week later I was feeling good. So I decided that I would attack some of the gardening work that I had been avoiding. I set to with vigour. Unfortunately half an hour or so into the work I attempted to lift a huge clod of soil.

I knew nothing in those days of correct lifting procedures. The inevitable happened and my back muscles locked in painful spasm. I was distraught.

Sick to the teeth with this continual affliction I had hoped that the chiropractor would have done the trick. I hope that I am not being derogatory, but clearly as far as I was concerned at the time the treatment was not up to the task. But at that time it was all I knew. And so the following day I trotted off to the clinic once again. The treatment table was one of those that can turn to a vertical position. The patient stands on a plate at the end, and then the table returns to a horizontal position with the patient on it. And so there I was once again on the treatment table with the practitioner manipulating my spine. This time I was very tense. My back was stiff and sore. I just had to grin and bear it. When he had finished working on my back he walked to my head to perform the 'whiplash' move. I was afraid of this. Petrified! In my mind I began to think of the damage that could be done. What this fellow was doing to me was not natural. However I had to let him get on with it. As I said, at that time this was all I knew that would give me relief from my pain.

The treatment was complete and the table was returned to a horizontal position. I attempted to lift my feet to walk but found that my back muscles had locked. Instantly I was in extreme pain. I was stuck to the spot. I could not move. I started to cry.

The practitioner summoned my wife who was waiting for me. She came into the treatment room, held my hand and gave me some words of comfort. Slowly and painfully I dragged my feet along the ground and out to the car waiting to take me home. Agonizingly I somehow managed to crawl into the back of the car. My wife drove me home. On the way I could feel every bump in the road. I was miserable, angry even. How could have I been so stupid to allow myself to be manipulated in such a way.

Eventually we arrived home. With great effort I manage to slide out of the car and painfully made my way into our house. I decided that I could not make it upstairs to the bedroom and settled onto the sofa in the TV room. My wife called the doctor, who, when she arrived, injected my back with a muscle relaxant.

Thus I lay on the sofa for the next three days. I had to pass water in a bottle and ask my wife to dispose of the contents for me. I was so ashamed. At the same time I wondered how I was going to get through the rest of my life living like a cripple. I cursed the chiropractor.

Apparently though, spinal manipulation has been used in various parts of the world and for thousands of years. Most of the practitioners seem to emanate from the USA where it does seem to be popular. Harvey Lillard was the man who had the first ever chiropractic adjustment. The first School of Chiropractic opened in

1898. Kansas was the first state to license Chiropractors in 1913. By 1941 the standards were set up to accredit Chiropractic schools. In 1944 the GI Bill of Rights made grants available for returning war veterans to study it. In 1972 the US Congress voted to make chiropractic available under Medicare. Now apparently there are about 50,000 Chiropractors in the USA with one in 15 Americans seeing a practitioner at least once a year. This is good and well. However my experience has convinced me that the name I have heard given to Chiropractors – 'Mr Crowbar' – may well be appropriate. I will leave you to make up your own mind.

What the visit to the Chiropractor did though was to open my mind to the fact that there might be alternatives that may just offer me some relief from my pain. And so I then decided that perhaps there might be some other form of therapy out there that might give me some help. It was suggested that I might try some acupuncture.

Accordingly I went to a local clinic and placed myself in the hands of a fellow. He asked me a few questions and once again I lay on a treatment table. He punctured my skin with a variety of needles. He then went off and left me for about twenty minutes. When he returned he asked me to dress and handed me a small bottle of brown liquid. I paid him quite a lot of money and left with an appointment for the following week. Quite frankly I did feel a bit better. However, again the relief did not last. I then found that this chap was quite happy to keep taking my money and asking me to return week after week. Perhaps I was silly to keep going to his clinic, but at the time I was clutching at straws.

Today he is a very rich man. However it made me sad to see people at his clinic with awful problems who were there for 'a cure!' I am sorry but 'cure' is a word that I would never offer to one of my patients. I am happy to try to offer help, give relief, and succour. But 'cure' never! As far as I am concerned from a Christian point of view the man who did the miracles died two thousand years ago and there hasn't been anyone like him since.

Acupuncture though is a very ancient art, part of the culture of China it originated 4000 to 5000 years ago. The term is derived from acus (needle) and puncture (puncture) and involves puncturing the skin with needles that go into the underlying tissue or even bone.

I understand that the traditional medicines of China have been persisted unchanged for thousands of years. The whole concept though is very alien to Western medicine. According to them the body is governed by the two essences of yin and yang, which are at once opposed and complimentary. Health is a perfect balance of the two. Disease is a disturbance of the balance between them.

Acupuncture is the insertion of needles at precisely determined points on the meridians (road maps in the body). This is supposed to encourage the blood to flow and moisten the bones and ligaments and lubricate the joints.

The trademark of classical acupuncture has a phrase that says "The superior physician is one who can successfully prevent diseases before they develop." The brief oriental view of pain is that it results primarily from stagnant or blocked Qi (life force). The needling point opens up the dam and allows the flow of energy through a meridian.

I have never studied Chinese medicine in any detail but I do have an interest in it. I must say that I do believe that it has its limitations. It is superb as a local anaesthetic. However, it was not the solution to my back problems. I found that the more treatment I had the less effective it was.

The other side of the coin though was a doctor who was out in the jungle in the Amazon some years ago. He was two days from the nearest village and a week away from hospital.

He was in a perilous state. He diagnosed that he had appendicitis: acute inflammation of the appendix, the commonest emergency in abdominal surgery. It is extremely dangerous in that the appendix may burst and cause a fatal spread of infection. This chap knew the danger he was in. However, in addition to being a doctor he was also a qualified acupuncturist. Thus by using his needles he administered his own anaesthetic and then set about removing his appendix. Then he sewed himself up and survived to tell the tale.

The Chinese have been practicing this form of medicine for all of these thousands of years, yet we only accepted it into the medical fraternity in the UK in 1977. In China the official government policy now calls for all hospitals to incorporate both Western and Eastern modalities. Hopefully we are not going to be too far behind them?

This led me to place my body in the hands of a little Japanese fellow I found in Glasgow. He laid me on his treatment table then proceeded to walk up and down my back with his bare feet.

Fortunately he was quite lightweight. However I was a fool to let him do what he did. I could have had something badly wrong with my back and perhaps he could have paralysed me. Thankfully it did not happen. However I had just one visit to his clinic.

My next port of call was at the home of a reflexologist. It is a focussed pressure technique, usually directed at the feet or hands. It is based on the premise that zones or reflex areas exist in the hands or feet that correspond to all organs, glands, and systems of the body. Stimulation of these reflex areas assists the body to biologically correct, strengthen and reinforce itself.

Apparently the ancient Egyptians as far back as 2500bc practiced it. The tomb of Ankhmahor, a physician of high esteem, at Saqqra is where the scene depicting the practice of reflexology is to be found.

The North American Indians have a philosophy that says: "Our feet walk on the earth and through this our spirit is connected to the universe. Our feet are in contact with the earth and the energies that flow through it." I was happy with the therapy offered, but once again it did little to help my back. I am saddened by the fact that since reflexology came to the UK it seems to have been diluted by in-fighting in the various Academies and Associations such that there are now several versions of it. I understand though that the UK government has suggested that they all bury the hatchet and come together under the one umbrella.

Over a number of years and all prior to finding my Holy Grail I experimented with visits to various 'back pain' clinics. Most of them gave me little in the way of relief. All were happy to take my money none the less. I learned as I went. Now I know that there are many forms of alternative medicine. 57 varieties at the last count!

These include such as Hypnotherapy, Meditation, Spiritual Healing, Tai Chi, Ayurveda, Alexander Technique, Cranio Sacral Therapy, Applied Kinesiology, Bonnie Pruden Miotherapy, Orthomolecular Medicine and such. Some of them take a bit of believing although I am sure that somewhere in their midst there will some gems that are of and will be in time to come of value to mankind.

Acupuncture it seems is the best of what is available especially as the World Health Organisation of the United States has identified more than 40 medical conditions effectively treated with acupuncture.

Despite its many 'claims to fame' sadly, I didn't find it good in helping my back pain, however, in all of this I am of the opinion that the Chinese have most to offer and thus in the years to come I will direct more and more of my studies in this direction. Apparently there are thousands of ancient Chinese scriptures as yet un-translated, so perhaps we all have lots to learn about how to help that infinite piece of intricacy – The Human Body!

Until that day comes by far the best of all alternative medicines, the one that saved me from years of misery and turned my life inside out is the therapy that I now practice and the one that you can all read about in the Holy Grail!

Chapter Twenty Three

DID GOD HAVE A BAD BACK

As the rich get richer and the poor get ever more used to life in the gutter, it does make you wonder if there is a God out there. Rich or poor, we all have bad backs. God makes no allowance in his calculation for wealth in health. We are all tarred with the same brush. That is of course assuming that you do believe in God. If you are pagan, an atheist or one whose soul has yet to be touched, then you might not agree with what I will write here. Nevertheless, I hope that you might understand the logic and the reason for writing such a chapter as part of this book.

In my opinion, belief in a God does not make you a bad person. If your God is important to you, you should be allowed to get on with your devotion without interference from others, worshiping your God in the way that your religion demands you do. Doing it in your own quiet way and certainly without any intrusion into your meditation, no matter what form it may take. It should matter not a jot that you decide to get down on a prayer mat at mid-day, use your compass to point the direction to Mecca or wherever and spend the next half hour bent double on the prayer mat. Perhaps you may be kneeling in a dimly lit chapel somewhere. The crease that you so lovingly put into your best cavalry twill pants destroyed. Knees aching! But the fact that you are able to sneak away from the office for ten minutes or so in your lunch break, to do what really matters is important. Spending a few minutes in solitude with your God is salient and serious. The little bit of time that you take talking to your mentor might just be the difference between sense, and nonsense as you struggle with daily life. A bit of calm amongst all of this hectic existence we all seem to lead.

It begs the question of course of "who is God?" Is it a he or a she or a thing that none of us will ever understand while we are alive, something that the human brain does not have the ability to comprehend? We cannot be alone in this vast universe.

It is just not possible. Out in the stratosphere there must be incredible matters that we will never get to grips with in any way of understanding. Over the centuries many of us have asked the same questions. What lies beyond the clouds? Does anyone live is out there? Is there another world just like ours yet situated just beyond the limits of ability of the communication equipment we use. Indeed in this other world are the inhabitants asking the questions that we do. It is frightening that we cannot find an answer. Too many of us though believe that there must be something out there, and so we call it God. We pray to it for answers to our worldly problems. We pray for relief from our back pain. It has become part of life.

Most of us will adopt whatever religion our parents had, and do so without question. We will quietly accept that they must have been right. We don't put our brains under too much stress trying to find the answer to the questions that pcrhaps we should be asking. It is better that way it would seem. In any case if you worked yourself into a frenzy trying to find the answer, trying to comprehend the un-comprehendible, your brain would explode, implode perhaps. And so our religion becomes part of our daily lives.

Accepting that this is so, most of us allow others to get on with their own version of the belief in a God. We don't interfere. At the same time we expect that others will give us the same space to indulge in whatever our religion demands. It does seem that what matters in religion is opinion. I have my opinion of what matters in my religion. However I don't shove this opinion into the face of anyone else. I keep it to myself. It is none the less important to me. Accepting that there is a God out there in that vastness which extends beyond our little planet, my religion should not matter a jot to anyone but me. It is personal and private to me and me alone. It is my own business. I don't care what religion you are. Yes of course I want you to be kind and care for your fellow human being. I am happy that you have faith in a religion.

My religion won't clash with yours. So please don't contradict mine. I will be kind to you, my fellow human being, in the same way that I expect you to be kind to me. That should be the basis of any religion. Sadly many a war that has been fought on this planet has started over some sort of religious argument. How stupid.

Despite this I get angry at people who poke their nose in where it is not welcome. What value do they place on knowing which religion I follow? Indeed what matter is it to them the religion of anyone. What I do or indeed what anyone does in their spare time is entirely up to them. As long as my belief does no harm, why should anyone bother? And yet too often I see examples of religious intolerance, especially in the work-place. Bigots, it would seem, are everywhere.

Externally we are all different. Fat, thin, tall, short we are all from a different mould. There is not one of us identical. Yet if we were to look at any human from any part of this hallowed planet, it would take forever to understand their culture, their language and all of the other things that make them what they are. But, strip the skin from the bodies, and what do we see, the same muscles, tendons, ligaments, nervous systems and hearts and lungs in all of them. Why, oh why, do we fight each other, when in reality under the skin, we are all brothers? We all have the same colour of organs, muscles and tissue. Yes the rich are rich and the poor are poor, but intrinsically we are all equal. We all have the same level of organisation and the same 11 systems (integumentary, skeletal, muscular, nervous, endocrine, cardiovascular, lymphatic, respiratory, digestive, urinary and reproductive) that God I believe gave us to make us the human beings that we are.

Thus it makes me mad that colour or creed will prevent people, real people with talent and a care for the work they do, from achieving the status in the work place they fully deserve.

The colour of your skin, or the church that you belong to, should have nothing to do with how successful you are in life, but often it does.

It troubles me when I see parents who have indoctrinated their offspring at an early age. Often I have seen the baby wear a tee-shirt with a message proclaiming the religion that they practice and the fact that they are willing and prepared to die for it. What for? The poor mites are only interested in their next meal. Religion, Bah! At any age below five who gives a toss. Clean nappies and ice creams are more of a priority. And yet many silly parents have it in their heads that just because their parents brought them up in a particular religion, then their own children have no choice in the matter. Pointless meaningless so-called religious rubbish forced into young minds that are never given a chance to develop an opinion.

I can see this in Catholic, Protestant, Muslim, Jew, or indeed any of the other multitudes of religions around the world. Today, the continuing conflicts in the Middle East, and the recent troubles in Northern Ireland to name but a few are examples of thoughtless senseless violence in the name of religion. Often the people fighting have little knowledge of why. They have never investigated why they will go out and kill someone because he went to the wrong school. How stupid and what a waste of human life.

It does make me sad to see that in all of this, the rich get richer. The people who make all of the rules in society today seem to be the ones with the most cash. Lesser mortals in this world, it would seem, have to do what they are told and have little choice. I am fortunate that I do have some say in how I lead my life.

But down in the basement the poor have to accept what is shoved in their face. In real terms, they are the ones who suffer.

Many financially prosperous people, it would seem, don't care about anything other than making yet more money, no matter how much they have. Of course there are a few nice ones who will give a slice of their income to charity, but most of the time it is the banks that benefit. Banks, according to many friends that I have, are dreadful nasty organisations. They could cancel the third world debt at a trice. It would make no difference to their profits. But greed, a sin in my book, won't let them do this. It would make you wonder if these people have any religion. Can they afford not to have one?

Life, as far as I am concerned, without belief in some kind of God scares the wits out of me. When you raise a finger, and point it at the sky, where does it all end? What is out there for goodness sake? How far could you travel if you had a rocket fast enough to take you there? What or who would you meet at the end of the journey? Would you come to a stop, bump into a brick wall? If you did, what would be on the other side - God and his entourage, who knows?

I don't want to be seen as being on my high-horse, but, not one of us has the answer, and yet we keep fighting each other for stupid reasons. "One two three what are we fighting for, don't ask me, I don't give a damn, next stop is Vietnam, five six seven open up the pearly gates, well there ain't no time to wonder why, yippee were all going to die," went the song in 1985. Country Joe and the Fish wrote it and sang it as a swipe at the Vietnam War. They could have it written about any war, anywhere. The lads in the trenches in the first or second world wars must have written similar songs. Just what is the point of war? Why do we have to have all of this needless heartache?

In all of this we have the issue of religious freedom and we have the horrendous abuse of human rights, often in oppressive regimes. Do we really have to have amputations and hangings, all in the name of religion? God in my opinion is a reflection of you. Thus if you are a nasty vengeful person you will have a nasty vengeful God. We fall out about the imaginary differences between us, but we fail to see the similarities. The sin of selfishness produces greed. Me, me, me, it would seem, is all we can think of. This of course produces the fear of loss, but that again is another story altogether. And in all of it the rich get richer. Many of them to this day are still living comfortable lives on the proceeds of the last war. Do they care and as I have said, do they have a God? Is he dispensable if you are rich?

It does seem to me that the young, indeed the middle-aged even give little regard to neither ethics nor the fact that indeed there may be a God to face at the end of their lives. Then as old age approaches and they begin to think that their allotted time scale on the planet is about to come to an end, they start to fear what may happen to their souls after they die? Then, perhaps they are afraid, and scared out of their wits. This is surely the time when we all have to admit that we should really have a God of some kind or another.

I have not had my allotted four score years and ten yet, or whatever number of years my God decides to give me, but at this time in my life I am afraid to die. I have made a sort of peace with my God in the hope that if he were to take me before I was ready to go then at least I have partially prepared for it. Not done the proper job, mind. But how many of us are prepared for death?

We all live our lives each day. Some of us do it in a quiet caring sort of way unobtrusively getting on with life as best we can. Poor! You bet. A lot of us are. There are though degrees of poor. Rich-poor and poor-poor! I remember a woman who lived in a town not far from me. She was going through a divorce. She petitioned the judge at the court hearing that her dog was in the habit of having nothing but the best. His daily intake of food consisted of smoked salmon, fillet steak and other opulent dishes. She went on to tell that she could never survive without her manservant pampering to her. Her delivery of groceries came from the most exclusive shop in town. She would be destitute if she could not afford to pay for the schooling of her little petal, the stuffed, overfed brat, and otherwise known as her darling daughter.

Considering the pleas from the woman, the judge in summing up advised that of course this woman was indeed entitled to a major chunk of her hard worked husband's income. And so, the (poor) woman settled down to a life of misery, or so she believed. What a bit of nonsense. The settlement awarded by the judge allowed more each week to the dog, than the honest working man in the adjacent village took home as a whole weeks pay.

In the end God has his way. We die. We are dust. The bank account, well it isn't much use when you have popped your corks. All the snivelling in courts to gain yet more riches is just a sham. When you are dead, the worms get you. They are the only ones who benefit. Of course one does have to ask, does a worm have a God? Are there rich worms and poor worms? Certainly I've seen big ones and little ones. Are they richer by size? Deep down in the ground do they have their own villas, central heating and all? And yet beside them, yes just yards away, the poor skinny worms are shivering from the cold, afraid that some big bird is coming to eat them. Perhaps it is extra for the subterranean hideaway that would keep them safe.

Oh God, are you out there? Why do we have to suffer? Me a poor worm with a bad back! It was OK until that great big lump of a gardener ran over me with his wheelbarrow this morning. Oh well, I suppose it is better than being eaten by a crow!

When I was a lad I used to stare up to the tops of the tall pine trees next to where I lived. The crows lived there. Nearer to God I thought. Not a bad back among them. Then I grew up, and realised that I was just as close to God as they were. I am sure though that amongst all of the squabbling over a bit of discarded food; there are the crows with bad backs. The poor things though can't complain. Their reward though will surely come, when they ascend to the big nesting ground in the sky.

This takes me back to when as children we had no choice. Our parents told us that we were one thing or another. We were dragged along to church or synagogue or mosque one or more days a week, whether we liked it nor not. At the establishment we had then to sit diligently and listen to the oration of some old fellow, long past his sell by date, prattling on in words that made little or no sense to us. There was no point to it. What did he know? The silly man, did he not realise were not listening. Gosh, the only thing that mattered was to get out of the place and get back to having some real fun with the friends we had left at play in the street.

A nurse once told me the tale about two boys who were in hospital, not with bad backs, but with broken femurs (the big bone from the hip to the knee). They had each been unfortunate to break this same bone which when healing, takes a long time. Usually you have to be in traction to make sure that it sets in the correct place. Anyway, these two wee boys were terrorising the other kids in the ward by asking if they were Catholic. If they were, they were given a hell of a time. Indeed these two horrible creatures were even terrorising the nurses.

One of the nurses decided that she had just about had enough of this disruption, and went off to check the records of the boys to see what religion if any they had. It turned out that one of them in fact was Catholic. The nurse returned and asked the lad if he knew that he was a Catholic. He retorted, "What is that?" In other words he didn't have a clue. Simply he had been indoctrinated at an early age, and believed what he had been told. The poor soul! What thoughtless parents he must have had.

However as we grow up, other thoughts enter the head. For example, are we alone in this universe? Is there any one else out there? Scientists reckon there is, but we are unable to find proof. I heard that they had found some evidence on the Moon. But the evidence could be only be interpreted as finding some tiny worms. 200 nanometers in size, (a nanometer is a billionth of a metre) the evidence was miniscule. Hardly big enough to be considered bacteria. Bacteria are so small that up to now we have found nothing smaller. However I understand that it would only take 8 days for bacteria to multiply and swamp a liquid planet, assuming that is that they had no enemies, and that it had an adequate supply of nutrients.

And so in our quest to find other living things in our solar system or indeed in any solar system, we have to ask if the evolution that we have enjoyed and which has given us life as we know it on this world evolved from these tiny worms. Perhaps one of the planets out there in the big vastness that we cannot understand is nothing other than a huge mortified lump of bacteria, stopped in time by a God who realised that indeed the evolution on Earth was a mistake. There it will stay waiting for us to find it someday when we have rockets fast enough to take us places we can only dream of at the moment. What we will make of it when this happens is anyone's guess. The only surety is that all of us here today, including those of with back pain won't be here to see it.

Statistically as far as I understand we cannot get anything smaller than a single cell. Yet this is what scientists are trying to find on any planet within our grasp. Just to prove that life exists or did exist, scientists thus are pulling their hair out to try to prove this theory, but the origin of life remains a mystery.

From what I can read I see that approximately 100 tons of planetary debris lands on the earth every day. Where does this come from? Indeed, how do scientists know that 100 tons lands every day? Statistics again! Who needs them?

And so what does all of this have to do with a back pain?

The situation as I understand it is that we have all been created in the likeness of our God. The perfect specimen that he would want us all to be! As a neonate we have our blueprint for life. We would all like to be perfectly fit humans, free from pain and suffering, and yet we are not. We have pain. Some of us have it in forms that others could not cope with. Many poor souls suffer with their pain in silence. They are the blessed of this earth. Others, the majority of us, whinge at the slightest discomfort!

There are lots of people like me who have had a life of having to cope with back problems. I suppose that thus afflicted we will all ask the same question. Why did my God make me like this? Why did he give me a bad back, with all of the associated pain and suffering? Is this my penance for being a bad boy in the last life? Was there a last life? Is this the only one we get? All these questions, and we don't have the answer to any of them. So, we just have to get on with the life that our God has given us, bad back and all. There is not much else we can do.

I consider myself to be very lucky in that despite the pain and suffering with my back over the years, I have managed to have some form of normality in life. I can now put my own socks on in the mornings. When I had my bad back I could not perform this simple task.

How many people out there in the big wide world would be happy just to be normal? How many of us take it for granted? We just don't know how lucky we are. Fortunately, in my mad scramble to find alleviation from my agony, I found the Holy Grail. It is a gift from God and a blessed relief from the torture that was my back pain. My health is not 100%, but 95% will do for me. It will see me happily through the rest of my life in the condition that it is in at the moment. If it is no worse that this I will be a happy chappie!

While we are on the subject of God, I suppose that we should say a few words about Mothers. What would we do without them? How many times have they been a support for our bad backs, and lots of other things too? When God was creating mothers, he had a difficult job. He had to give them quite some specification. They had to be able to run on cold tea and left over food. They had to have a kiss that could cure anything from a bad back, to a broken leg, or the disappointment of bad homework results. They had to have many pairs of eyes. They had to survive when all around them was falling apart. In all of this though, never would they complain of a bad back.

Often bent over the kitchen sink washing piles of dishes, or bathing a child with dirty knees, or bending to pick up yet another heavy load of washing for the drying line, or scrubbing the floor, their backs took all the punishment. My mother did all of these things without a word of thanks. When we were young my brother, sisters and I must have been ungrateful children. My mother's poor back must have been strained to breaking point, yet not once did she complain. My mother was just like many others out there. She never complained and just got on with things.

When she departs for the big kitchen in the sky I am sure that she will join all of the other mothers up there where God will look after all of them forever after. Like all mothers she will have her just reward, and rightly so.

My bad back, my pain and suffering pale into insignificance when compared with what my mother has had to cope with in her life. She is still with us today. It is only now that I am older that I am beginning to appreciate how much I owe her for what she did for me as I grew up. I just hope that I get the chance to show her the thanks she so richly deserves. So all of you out there reading this little book, rather than feeling sorry for yourself, moaning about your problems, think about your mother, and what she did for you.

But life, just like a party, has to end sometime. Ultimately we are all dead men, but how we lived our lives is how we will be remembered. A man I knew lived in my town, just down the road from where I reside. He was a member at my church. He attended regularly. As far as I could see he was as kind a man as anyone could ever meet. I knew that he loved his garden and that he spent hours working in it, cultivating the produce that he would cheerily disperse to poor folk who needed it. In turn the gardening gave him back pain. Yet he never complained. A nicer fellow you couldn't have met. When he died I went to his funeral service. It was my joy to be there. In life he lived by the values of the Gospel. His coffin was covered with a white pall. A sign of his baptismal garment, and the Christian dignity it bestowed upon him.

It was his belief and mine that the ties of love, friendship and affection, which knit us all together, do not unravel with death. Confident that God remembers the good we have done in life I was happy that he would gather him up to Him, now that he was dead. In our grief he had returned to God. The God of love is always ready to hear our cries: a God that would forgive this man the sins of his life and grant him a place of happiness, light and peace in the kingdom of glory forever. In the arms of God bad backs don't exist.

As for this man, he was like grass; he flowered like the flower of the field; the wind blew and he was gone, and this place never sees him again. Before he went though, he had forgiven those who had trespassed against him. How many of us could do this?

In sacred Scripture we read; "blessed are those who have died in the Lord; let them rest from their labours for their good deeds go with them".

I hope that you don't find it strange that I have written about God, in a book that is about back pain. In this chapter I haven't answered the question posed. I can't, as I simply don't know if God indeed had a bad back, or not. I have though written the words in the book in the hope that together we might be able to overcome some of the problems that we have in the world today. Back pain hurts many of us and takes away much of the joy of living, but in real terms it is nothing when compared to the other troubles that we see on a daily basis.

In anger we constrict the muscles of our face. It takes more to frown than to smile. I am sure that our backs suffer in the same way. Much of what I have written over the last few pages may be seen as a rant. Nonetheless I have the feeling that there is just too much injustice in the world today. I apologise if I have caused any upset. I mean no harm. We could all do our bit to make this planet a better place. I just hope that I can do my bit to leave this world a better place than I found it.

I would like to end this bit of this wee story by giving you an extract from a hymn that I know, and sometimes sing as I drive my car. I apologise to whoever wrote it. I do ask their permission to print these words. I hope that in the context of what I have written they will give it from above.

Make me a channel of your peace.
Where there is hatred, let me bring your love.
Where there is injury, your pardon Lord.
And where there's doubt, true faith in you.

Make me a channel of your peace.
Where there's despair in life, let me bring you hope.
Where there is darkness only light and
sadness ever joy.

Make me a channel of your peace.
It is in pardoning that we are pardoned,
In giving to all men that we receive, and
In dying that we're born to eternal life.

Chapter Twenty Four

THE HOLY GRAIL

When I started my research for this book I was aware that there have been many people who have but one book in them. It will be their life story. It may perhaps be sad. It may well be hilarious. It may be a best seller or indeed it could just be a whole load of rubbish. Nevertheless, for that particular person it will be an achievement.

In writing a book there is a lot of tough work. Nothing is accomplished easily. But any writing, good or bad should be cherished. It is one's innermost thoughts put down on paper. There is a great deal of hard graft in it. There has been in this one and I have written this book with a 'Holy Grail' at the end of it for a purpose.

It has been my intention to give these thoughts, words and considerations to you in a sensible manner. I have led you through some of the bits of my life. In doing so I have tried to explain in layman's terms what can happen to someone who suffers from back pain. Thus I hope that you may now understand some of the principles of back pain in just a little more detail. I trust that I have managed to write the words sensibly and I hope that by reading and absorbing the contents of the book it might help you to resolve your own back pain.

The preceding chapters have each been written for a purpose. They are written in ordinary language that I am hopeful every one of you can understand. My tips are given to help prevent your own back pain and are written as part of my experience with back pain, a pain that at times was excruciating. Now finally, in this book we have, with apologies to all of the best writers out there, reached our Holy Grail. Much like Arthur and his Knights of the Round Table, we have reached our zenith and achieved our goal.

Although this book tells lots of stories about me and other people that I know who have suffered with back pain, I have held this part of it purposely until the end. Perhaps after reading this chapter you may go back to the beginning and read the book again. Certainly I hope that you will read it for reference. Hopefully you will follow the advice about drinking water, exercising, lifting and sitting, etc; indeed I will be disappointed if you don't.

What indeed is the Holy Grail? Does it in fact exist or is it just a simple way to end the tale? Am I allowing matters to drift as in fact I don't have an ending to the book? Well the answer to all of this is No! The Holy Grail is Bowen Neural Therapy. I should explain how I found it or indeed it found me. Undeniably it has been my saviour.

During the earlier years of life I had been brainless. I didn't look after my body. Health was not an issue. All that mattered was each day as it appeared in front of me. I gave no thought to the future. Because of my stupidity my back suffered and in time it got worse. My muscles on many an occasion went into spasm that was agonising. It often happened for no reason. Yet when it did it floored me.

I was experiencing real pain. At times it was so painful that it seemed to me like the torture that some poor soul on the operating table undergoing surgery without anaesthetic would suffer. I was so depleted that I considered suicide. My very existence was at such a low ebb that I had nothing to look forward to but a life of painful discomfort. Mobility by wheel chair seems absurd when I think about it now, but when all you have in front of you is pain and suffering, it was a reality staring me in the face. Indeed I could begin to imagine why people would want to join the euthanasia society. I was nearly one of their members.

I experimented with all sorts of orthodox medicine. I allowed cortisone injections in my spine. What a fool I was; if only I had known then what I know now, I would never have let the orthopaedic surgeon near me. Many of the footballers that played for England in the 1966 World Cup Final had injections of cortisone pumped into the tissue in their knees just to keep them going and did so, on a regular basis. In those days the medics looked upon it as some sort of miracle cure. What they did not appreciate was that the cortisone destroyed the tissue in the players' knees, which in turn wore away the cartilage. (Cartilage reduces friction between bony surfaces). When it was gone, the players were left with bone rubbing on bone. As a result these players now have chronic arthritis and from what I have read now find even walking difficult. What a price to pay for success! Let us hope that the Lord forgives the doctors and surgeons who prescribed it. Thankfully, I had just two injections of this horrible substance. (See Bibliography: Managing Injuries in Professional Football)

I believe there is a place for physiotherapy and other forms of alternative medicine that have been properly researched, but an awful lot of what is available in the alternative and orthodox medicine world is brutal. Manipulation hurts. Surgery had to be out of the question. With a success rate of about 25%, just thinking about it frightened the life out of me. The possibility that I might well end up paralysed and in a wheelchair after an op that 'went wrong' was not worth the risk. Many a sleepless night I mulled over the pros and cons. This and many other thoughts often ran through my brain.

By reading this book I hope that you can learn from me and steer clear of some of the 'quacks' that are out there. Thankfully the Government in the UK have started to put things in order. In November 1999 (See Bibliography: Select Committee on Science and Technology) the House of Lords published a report.

It advised that the British public spent around £500m on alternative medicine in that year.

In recent years there has been an explosion of it in the country, yet with the National Health Service in such turmoil it is hardly surprising. I have often stated that we should call it the 'National Sick Service' as people only go to the doctor when they are ill. Nonetheless this report demands that all forms of alternative medicine will have to raise their standards to an acceptable level and it gives a time limit in which they have to do it. This can only be to the benefit of the people in the UK. I just hope that the Government completes the task. Allowing that the report was published six years ago, it is disappointing that since then the progress has been slow.

In the early days of my back pain I spent a lot of time at my GP looking for whatever help he could offer. Pain comes without much notice. It appears least when you expect it. Thus hurt as I would be, yet living in this modern fast track world I would often phone my GP at short notice demanding an appointment. My doctor works in the same remorseless world as we do and arriving at his surgery there was no immediate attention. I had to queue and join the line of other poor unfortunates that had presented themselves with all sorts of ailments, real or imagined.

Eventually it would be my turn. The problem then was that while I would want half an hour to fully explain what was troubling me, the doctor had just seven minutes of time to give me. He was under pressure to churn me through the system. In consequence in that limited period he was lucky to get half of the story of my misery. The upshot was that like most doctors mine had little choice but to prescribe a box of pills to mask the pain. Making an attempt at understanding the root cause of the problem in the limited time that he had to give me invariably resulted in the expensive 'quick fix'! The end result was, that without doubt in a short space of time I would find myself once again back at his office looking for yet more pills. The cost to the nation, well, who knows?

To be fair not all doctors have this attitude, but sadly it would have to be my opinion that the majority do. If you have a kind enduring and understanding doctor these days, as I now have, you are just lucky. This of course is not so if you are blessed and have been fortunate to find a Bowen Neural Therapist.

How I found BNT or indeed how it found me is a story that started about ten years or so ago. I was, at the time, drifting from one so-called treatment to another desperately searching for something, which would get to the bottom of my back pain. In those days I would have drunk a can of vinegar with two worms in it, every day, if it had eased my trauma. I would have washed myself in acid. In the process, stupidly, I accepted in good faith all sorts of bad advice. There I was stumbling from one crisis to another. In between I was clutching at straws. Daily life became a trial. It was hard work just to do ordinary things.

I was a member at a really good golf course, but as time went on I engaged in the recreation I loved less and less. Just about every time I played a round of golf or even just a few holes at times I would experience some kind of back pain. Many a day I could not finish my game of golf and always the morning after I would be as stiff as a board. My back muscles would often go into spasm.

The chapter about giving up golf (accepting that I have returned to participate as a better and altogether healthier player) tells about one of my most horrible moments. All in all I was in a sorry state. Worse though is the fact that no one believed that I had a bad back. If you have a broken leg you have a plaster cast as evidence. If you have an operation on a stomach ulcer you have the surgeon's scar to prove the emergency operation. Then you can get sympathy. With back pain the normal retort is "Oh yes, we believe you" when in fact people are really thinking that you are just using it as an excuse to have a few days off work.

Having to give up golf was the hard bit. I am not all that

proficient at the game, but there are times when I can hit the ball as well as anyone. For lack of better words "it was really doing my brain in". I was morose. Of course I never gave up hope. I always had to look forward to the day when indeed I might find a 'cure' no matter how miniscule the chance of this seemed.

One year as Christmas was approaching; I was a bit down in the dumps. I seemed to spend all of my time working hard to earn enough to pay the bills and the mortgage for the lovely house that we lived in. I have always enjoyed some of the better things in life, which of course included the cost of paying the subscription to my golf club. Thus I thought that it would be good if I could find some way to earn some extra cash and so I thought, why not write a book about my trials and tribulations? It would not have a happy ending, but it would be a true story of my life. I would end in a wheel chair!

While writing the book I was always aware that I might be wasting my time. I might not be able to find an understanding publisher. Thankfully as you can see I have managed to get the book in print. The task was not an easy one but I am one of life's survivors and I don't give up very easily. It had not been many years since I could hardly type a word. I can well remember my first bumbling efforts, pushing the keyboard of my first ever computer to one side of the desk and typing with one finger. However, with the view that I will always try to make some money wherever I can, and as a qualified quantity surveyor working in the construction industry, I had a deal of experience in the subject of house building. So I decided to write to a magazine that was dedicated to explaining the efforts of people who had built their own homes, and offer my services. I was pleased when they asked me to go down to London to meet in their office.

I was delighted when at the end of the interview they asked me to write the articles about homes that were being built in Scotland and the north of England.

So, I worked for a national publisher with many fine titles in their stable. In the process they sent me to interview the people who had built their own homes. I put to words the story of how they did it and joined it to the pictures taken by the photographer who accompanied me. My name was in print, and I earned some much needed cash. I was a proud man.

With some of the earnings from the magazine articles I went to my golf club, where I knew there was a nice selection of good quality goods, to purchase a sweater for my wife. The professional in the shop at the club asked me why he had not seen me hitting a golf ball for a long time. I had to tell him that I just couldn't. My back was knackered.

The golf course that has me as one of its members has an elevated status in the golfing world. The final qualifying rounds for the Open Championship are played over it when the Open comes to Scotland. It hosts other prestigious competitions. The consequence of this is that it is difficult to secure a membership. When I first applied 35 years or so ago, it took about 10 years on the waiting list before I was admitted. Being so difficult to gain entry in the first place was probably the reason why I was reluctant to give up one of the things in life that I really cherished.

If I gave up my membership, I would be unlikely to regain it. The waiting list today is longer than it was when I first applied for membership. As a result I had continued to pay my subscription, yet for a number of years all I could do was watch from the club-house window as my fellow members enjoyed the game that my physical difficulty prevented me from enjoying.

The professional listened to my saga with a sympathetic ear. Then he told me something that was to change my life. He suggested that some of the lads at the golf club had gone to a fellow who gave them some form of therapy. It seemed that it resolved back problems. I agreed that I would give it a go, but I was sure that it would be just another waste of time and money. Nonetheless, off I toddled and made an appointment. I arrived at the clinic, which presented itself as a place for 'the treatment of sports injuries'. I entered with caution. The last thing that I wanted was manipulation or needles sticking into me. I had endured enough pain.

I told my story to the fellow. He seemed a nice man. He did not take many notes. Quickly he had me on his treatment table. I lay face down. He made some puzzling movements across my skin in a variety of places. However, it did not hurt. After a while he asked me to turn onto my back. I did this gingerly. Attempting this movement had often been something which would knock my back muscles into painful spasm. In reality it had happened sometimes when I turned in my sleep, awakening me with a jolt. Anyway, I managed to do what he wanted and he continued with the treatment.

After about thirty or forty minutes he announced that for that session the treatment was complete. He was going to ask me to rise from the table. He slid his hand under my shoulder and made to lift me. I shouted "Whoa". Immediately I flushed with sweat. What he was asking me to do was a simple task for someone who was fit, but something that I, a back pain sufferer, had not attempted for years. I asked him to pause for a minute until my brain stopped swirling and I stopped sweating. I explained my fear. He gave me some words of comfort and told me that it would not hurt. I put my trust in him and fairly quickly he sat me up. I took some deep breaths thankful that my back muscles were not in spasm. I dressed and went home. I could feel something funny going on inside my body but I was not sure what it was.

I returned to this man's clinic at seven day intervals. After each visit I could feel that things were getting better and better. I was eventually, gingerly at first, able to put my own socks on. I asked him what treatment he was giving me. Although he did not advertise the fact, he told me that he practised a number of modalities and with them some Bowen therapy that he had used to help me. I was intrigued. Life was beginning to get back together. Back pain and all that went with it was starting to look like it could soon be something of the past. My therapy continued for a number of weeks. I had to pay, but I was happy that after all this time; at last I had stumbled on something that was helping, rather than the usual so-called therapist who was more interested in taking my money or indeed the doctor giving me a pill to mask the pain, this therapy was actually addressing the problem.

I started to quiz the fellow about the therapy that he practiced. Was there a book about it? Where could I find out more about it? He told me that in fact there were no books on the subject of his therapy. He only had technical manuals that I would not be able to understand. However, he astounded me by suggesting that I should perhaps consider going off to learn the therapy myself. I protested that I had trained and qualified as a quantity surveyor. I was fascinated by his suggestion.

And so I went home and announced to my wife that I was going to become a therapist. She thought that I was nuts. In spite of this, I was determined and so I got hold of the head office number and applied to join the Bowen Association UK which is associated to the Bowen Therapy Academy of Australia (BTAA). I began my studies in Leicester in England.

I had to travel down on Friday evenings after work and study with a lovely group of enthusiastic people who were as keen to learn as I was. It was fascinating, but awfully hard work.

A major problem was that I did not come from a medical background. All of the other people on the course had some sort of medical history. They were either doctors or nurses, or midwives or they had trained in other forms of alternative medicine. They knew how the body worked while I had not much of a clue. So I had the task of learning all that I could about anatomy and physiology, get myself a first aid practicing certificate, complete my Bowen studies and do all of this while I held down my day job as a quantity surveyor.

The Bowen studies continued in Edinburgh which saved travelling to Leicester. I had a new tutor here who was puzzled at some of the work that I had been taught by the instructor in Leicester. However, he seemed to be able to iron out the intricacies and little by little my knowledge improved. It did leave me to wonder why I had been taught differently by two people who were supposed to be 'singing from the same hymn sheet'. It further gave me an insight into the complexities and politics that seem to cause such controversy in associations such as this.

All of this opened my eyes to another side of medical life that I just did not know existed. In my chapter on other alternative therapies I have explained that I did not know that there were so many of them. I should admit that until I got involved in Bowen I was a complete sceptic. Alternative medicine was all but hocus-pocus. Yet as a convert I was now ferreting away trying to glean as much information about anything in health care that was complimentary and alternative.

In my studies I have come to the conclusion that some complimentary and alternative medicine is junk. Bits of it are awfully difficult to believe. But, in the midst of all of this debris, there are some therapies which demand closer inspection. The problem that I can see is that they are not at all properly regulated. It seems that the hobby housewife can spend a couple of weekends on a course and immediately hang a bit of worthless paper on the wall professing that indeed she is now an expert in her subject. The public are sadly gullible and simply don't ask the questions that they should do to prove that indeed the woman has completed a structured and methodical tutorage that had an examination at the end of it. The certificate given should explain much like a university degree the level of competence.

In addition to the certificate on the wall, any prospective patient should ask if the therapist has an anatomy and physiology diploma and ask further if indeed he/she does in fact understand the complexities of the human body and the reason why people are in pain. Or, as I suspect, is the person just out to make a bit of money and in the process perhaps do more harm to the patient than good? The words of course directed to the hobby housewife apply equally to men in the same category.

In the depths of despair, with my back muscles in spasm when I was at my wits end, I suppose that I was often clutching at straws and many a time placed my body in the hands of such a person offering any form of relief. In times like this we can be very foolish. Hindsight of course is a great thing.

In addition to training as a nurse, my wife Sheila had qualified some years ago as a clinical aromatherapist. Massaging with oils and having men as well as women as patients did not go down well with me. It was a dirty business I thought, with sexual overtones even. What an idiot I now realise I was.

About a year or so after I was converted to Bowen I lay in bed one night. As I lay, I subconsciously rubbed my feet together. They were itchy. I had Athletes Foot (not that I knew at the time). I had tried all sorts of lotions, potions and powders without success. Sheila was fed up and angry that she was being awakened from her sleep.

She sat up and said that she would make me something to stop the itching. She made some lotion with her oils and I applied it to my feet. I suppose that I was hardly surprised that it worked. The itching stopped. I followed her application instructions to the letter. The itching has never returned. For this and other reasons I am indeed a convert to alternative medicine. My wife of course is happy that she gets a good night's sleep.

I mentioned that I am pleased that the Government has decided to take steps to regulate alternative therapies. There are just too many unscrupulous people out there happy to take the money from the public. They give very little in return. Thus the government acknowledging this have decided to act. In doing so hopefully they will cut out the cranks and the unscrupulous operators!

What it has asked in the report of 1999 is that the fragmented bits of any of these therapies must join together as one association. They must train their therapists to an acceptable standard, have them regimented and recorded and insist on some form of continuous professional assessment much as doctors have to do.

Sadly there are fragmented versions of Bowen in different parts of the world. The Bowen Therapy Academy of Australia was the original. I am happy still to be a member, although for how long this lasts remains to be seen. Now and again we have had words. Being a bit of a revolutionist I don't agree with all of the rules. At times my relationship with the Academy has been tenuous.

Anyhow, as they say about the University student: no matter how much he may disparage the University they cannot take the University degree from him. Thus, as I have the certificate, I shall continue to use the letters BTAA after my name.

Why, you may ask, are there fragmented versions? The answer may well be simply financial greed. I quickly came to appreciate in many of the alternative therapies I have studied that the originator was often a kind gentle person whose only aim was to spread his or her own gospel. Simply making people better the aim, they often they look for little financial return. Rarely are they businessmen or women. Financial success is the last thing on their mind. As far as I can see Tom Bowen (the originator of Bowen Therapy) was such a person. But people such as this are rare and at times are at the mercy of others who recognise this and manipulate matters for their own gain. They appropriate the idea and with just a few alterations to the original menu, that at times have little substance, they set up their own substitute version of the therapy. You can draw your own conclusion as to whether or not their aim is simply to make money. On that I will not comment. The result inevitably is fragmentation. It does little for the decent therapies that are out there. Thus the government has demanded the houses are put in order.

We are lucky here in the UK to have a man who has more than a passing interest in alternative medicine in all its varied forms. The Prince's Foundation for Integrated Health was formed at the personal initiative of HRH the Prince of Wales, who is now its President. The Foundation takes the view that the quality of the treatment combined with public safety must take the highest priority, and with this I can only agree. The primary reason is to safeguard the pubic, and while again I accept this as a main concern I can see that the benefit to the practitioner. Their status will be enhanced as the public begin to perceive the improved standards in a profession that is still regarded by many as being a form of prestidigitation.

Professions that have been asked to join together in this consultation document and eventually to combine in one regulatory body are: Alexander Technique, Aromatherapy, Bowen Technique, Cranial Therapy, Homeopathy, Massage Therapy, Naturopathy, Nutritional Therapy, Reflexology and Yoga Therapy.

The professional associations for acupuncture and herbal medicine have already established their own regulatory working groups. Allowing that many practitioners are multi-disciplinary it is obvious that setting up this federal regulatory structure can only be for the good.

HRH Prince Charles is a good fellow. Much the same age as I am he has a liking for alternative medicine and does some sabre-rattling from time to time to remind the establishment of its existence. I know that his heart is in the right place. I do though feel that he gets poor advice. Perhaps one day I will get the opportunity to speak with him and give him my words of wisdom.

From what I can see from the consultation paper the therapists will have to prove that they have studied their own modality to a recognised level. Diplomas in Anatomy and Physiology must be the norm. Therapists must be able to understand the workings of the human body. In addition, as doctors have to, they will be expected to attend regular refresher courses. Continuous professional assessment! Examination boards will be assumed to have a reasonable standard that in turn will set assessments to stretch the therapist to the limit. Knowledge of their therapy must be unbounded. As far as I am concerned this is the only way forward. If alternative medicine ever wants to get anywhere it must in the eyes of the public be seen to be self-regulating and with this I can only agree.

In the 1999 report the government asked another very important question in that it requests that we prove the efficacy of our modalities. To do this it is suggested that we will have to conduct clinical trials. Clinical trials require a large sample size. In simple terms this means that big numbers of people will be tested to prove that the therapy works. The methodology of how this is done is not for this book but suffice to say this is the way that medicine has proved itself over the years.

The Bowen Academy of Australia has gone a little way down the prescribed route to satisfy all of these demands. In addition, I can only hope that they will begin the task of repairing the fragmentation of the original therapy developed by Tom Bowen, but without the politics that currently envelope and upset its workings.

BTAA have already completed and published the results of a number of small-scale studies. These are:

- The Psycho-physiological Effects of the Bowen Technique Therapy by Ashley G Pritchard, Swinburne University, Melbourne. Department of Psychophysiology – 1993.

- A gentle hands on healing method that affects Autonomic Nervous Systems as measured by heart rate variability and clinical assessment – Jo Anne Whitaker MD, Patricia Gilliam Med., MSN. Douglas B Seba PhD.

- A potential treatment for Fibromyalgia – Doug Seba PhD.

- Evaluation of Bowen Technique in the treatment of Frozen Shoulder – Dr. Bernadette Carter – University of Central Lancashire. UK.

Other studies proposed are:

- Royal Lancaster Infirmary, England, Women and Children's Unit. The study will investigate antenatal problems in pregnancy, such as morning sickness, heartburn, low back pain, symphyseal pain, and breast discomfort.

- Chattham Memorial Hospital, North Carolina, USA. This study will compare outcomes between patients who received standard modalities and those treated with Bowen Therapy for acute and chronic patients that have not responded to traditional treatment. Apparently a number of symptoms will be examined.

Completing the task of making the modality evidence based will take some time and accepting that the current studies are small-scale, at least a start has been made. However, Scotland has led the world in medical research many a time and, taking matters into consideration with respect to the work that has been done in the Academy, I decided that it was time to take the bull by the horns and do something about it myself.

I treat a number of people who suffer with, amongst other symptoms, Multiple Sclerosis. The therapy that I practice is known as Bowen Neural Therapy (BNT). It is a blend of the original Bowen from Australia, Neural Touch that I learned from Gene Dobkin in the USA (I will talk about this later on) and other matters of research and conclusions that I have come to myself. I don't mix it with other modalities such as Reiki or any of the more 'weird' modalities, but I do have an interest in physiology and in particular myofascial dysfunction that perhaps has much to do with back pain.

There isn't much point in trying to explain myofascial pain dysfunction syndrome as it is a controversial, fundamentally outmoded term that has been considered to mean a syndrome largely of muscular origin, a complex psychophsiological phenonomenon, or a syndrome due to occlusal mechanics. Suffice to say that it is something that again is too complex for this book, yet if you care to have a look at my web-site (details at the end of the book) I will be happy to share the results of my research with you, and explain the illogical bits written in terms that you can understand.

Additionally, I have trawled the world looking at everything and anything in the medical world that has anything to do with back pain. In consequence I hope that I have acquired knowledge from one person or another that I have studied with, and in all of this, I hope, I have improved my understanding of the human body. In turn I trust that this makes me a better Bowen Neural Therapist.

In the process of all of this, it would seem that I able to offer help to some of the unfortunate people in Scotland who suffer with Multiple Sclerosis (MS). Many that endure such a burden are on a slippery slope to nowhere. Often they have experimented with drugs of one kind or another. Recently I have met some who have gone abroad to take some stem cell treatment. Despite the high cost of much of this, there seems to be such limited success in controlling the symptoms of MS. However, a year or so ago, accepting that Bowen and its derivatives was able to do at least something to help this horrible affliction, I encouraged a number of other Bowen practitioners that I know to join me in a study.

At the time we knew little about the complexities of such work and perhaps more to the point even less about the variety of symptoms that affect people who suffer with MS. Very soon we came to the conclusion that we had over-reached ourselves.

For a variety of reasons the group disbanded and I put everything on the back-burner affirming that, at one day in the future I would return to complete the work necessary in such a study, no matter how complex. Needless to say the days of inactivity in relation to this turned into weeks and the weeks into months.

Then one day I decided that it was time to take matters forward. I made a pact with myself that I would try to convince the NHS that the examination of the therapy that I practice to prove its efficacy would not just be beneficial to patients, but additionally could save the NHS money.

I am fortunate to have a number of doctors and surgeons and other academics who come to my clinic for treatment. They are all interested in my research programme. One of the academics in particular will often discuss matters with me. In conversation one day I explained the dilemma that I had with the MS research and told him that I had decided to commence with a study at the other end of the spectrum where the efficacy would be simpler to prove and that in fact I would look at how BNT is able to help patients who suffer from nocturnal enuresis (bed wetting).

Countless people wet the bed, yet it would seem that this is a bigger problem than many families will ever admit to. A lady patient once told me a story about her son (lets call him Robbie) who could not go to a birthday party at the weekend as it would involve a sleepover. Robbie's mum had to make the excuse that the family was going away for the weekend and as such Robbie wouldn't be able to go to the party. In reality the truth was that there would be a risk that Robbie would wet the bed and in consequence the parents would be ashamed to admit that their son had perpetrated such an act. The woman used the excuse as the reason why Robbie could not attend.

She was happy when I was able to help her son and after some treatment, help him cease the bed-wetting. At least then Robbie would indeed be able to enjoy his sleep-over with his chums. I treat this problem on a regular basis. I have a good success in finding resolve to a difficulty that affects not just children but older people just the same. My success isn't 100%. Nothing is in life. I have never quantified my success rate. Nonetheless, I would think that it is perhaps as high 80%. However, when suggesting the idea for such a study to the academic he suggested to me that it was the wrong subject to commence with. Nocturnal enuresis is not life threatening; it doesn't cost the country any money and it is "not fashionable" are the words that he used to convince me.

I protested that it was a simple procedure to evaluate. Either you do or you don't wet the bed. There is no in between. Nonetheless my academic patient and friend suggested that it would be best to consider commencing with a study that would examine the efficacy in relation to people who suffer with back pain. Thousands of people in the UK suffer with the problem. The cost to industry in financial terms runs to many millions of pounds. Doctors don't have any answers to such a problem other than to dole out yet more analgesics that simply mask the pain and don't address the problem. And so I accepted his advice.

Setting up such a study demands a number of issues be addressed. A relationship has to be built with a university that has an interest in alternative medicine and who will be prepared to work with someone like me. There is the burden of having to find the funds not just to pay the cost of treating the 60 or so people (on the pilot study) that will attend for treatment but also to fund the university in respect of all of the academic work that will be necessary.

I would have to write the protocol before presenting it to the Ethics Committee at the General Medical Council (GMC) (or the Ethics Committee of the GMC local to me) prior to actually starting the work. Then of course I would have to monitor the work as it proceeds, write up the results and publish a paper at the end.

Finding a university that would cooperate was a difficult task. I wrote to many. Most wouldn't answer my letters. Some quite frankly were elitist and frowned on the thought of undertaking a study that wasn't part of general medicine or more importantly supported by a drug company. For months I trawled through one university, college and centre of learning after another. In the process I had many meetings and trips that offered yet one false hope after another. However everyone has to have a bit of luck in life and indeed I did in finding an organisation that works at Edinburgh University.

It is thus with thanks to Dr. Siobhan Jordan and the work that she did for me that I was able in turn to make contact with Napier University who have now agreed to discuss collaboration in my study. I have written a few words about Interface as follows, just in case there is a budding scientist reading this book (albeit one who suffers with back pain!).

Interface – the knowledge connection for business offers a free service to companies. More details can be found here www.interface-online.org.uk

- Many companies do not know that innovative solutions to help their business grow can be developed with University assistance. Interface is the first point of contact to help make this happen as it is representing all of Scotland's universities.

- Interface can easily identify and facilitate introductions to potential academic collaborators across all of the Scottish Universities by finding the relevant expertise to meet business needs

- Interface overcomes the challenge facing companies in understanding what is available or who to contact in Scottish Universities for R&D or expertise capabilities

Since the initial help from Interface, I have had a number of meetings with Napier. The plan (subject to a number of conditions) is that they allow me a studentship that will permit me to study for an MSc in Health Science. In time this should lead to a PhD. It seems a very tall order. However, accepting that I wish to leave this planet a better place than I found it and having a wish to help my fellow human beings, I am quite prepared for the nights when I will have to burn the midnight oil. Research is an 'old boys club' and I will have to learn the language.

In the Masters degree I would hope to be able to prove the efficacy of the therapy (or indeed disprove) by completing (with the help of the University) and publishing the results of a number of research modules. This is my plan for the future and perhaps will give me more to write about in the next book.

The originator of Bowen, the late Tom Bowen, had a clinic in Geelong in Victoria State in the south of Australia. His work has stood the test of time and as the years have gone by the number of practitioners who use his methods or abridged versions of it has grown. From Tom's original relationship with Oswald Rentsch (I will talk about Oswald later on) has grown the Bowen Therapy Academy of Australia.

I was privileged in March 2000 to be a speaker at the International Conference in Brisbane, Australia. The conference was fascinating and lasted for almost a week, during which time we had a host of good speakers who spoke on a variety of medical topics. At the end of the conference on the Saturday evening we had a gala dinner. There I met René Horwood who had worked as Tom's secretary and confidant. I shared a glass of her favourite Australian wine with her and listened as she spoke about her happy memories working with Tom.

During the conversation she told me that while Tom worked

with his patients performing his 'little miracles' he used to say to her "René – this works, but I don't know how it works!" He described his wonderful metaphysical concept as a 'Gift from God'. I have such happy memories of the conference. As with most of the people that practice Bowen (in its various forms) I never met the great man, as he died in 1982. Yet, Tom was the catalyst for much that has happened in the alternative medicine world since then. For all that he has done, and the seeds that he sowed in others (such as me) and other more eminent people, it would have to be my opinion that he now deserves to be in Heaven. Up there, perhaps he is sorting God's bad back?

Without him and the wisdom that he had to develop this technique I can assure you that I would not be the healthy person that I am today. Thus my tale has reached the point where I must tell you just a little about the wonderful man himself. The man, whose teaching led me to my Holy Grail.

The story of the life of Tom Bowen has never been recorded. Some bits of the history are a bit hazy and what I have written here has been gleaned from Gene Dobkin, Oswald Rentsch, and Rene and from the few others who studied with Tom. I apologize for any inaccuracies.

Thomas Ambrose Bowen lived from 1916 to 1982. It seems that he was intuitive and gifted. He devoted his lifetime to developing his original technique. He was described as insular and non-communicative, nonetheless his teachings have survived and prospered. Apparently he studied medicine prior to World War II with the intention, as far as we know, of becoming a doctor. The war intervened and he was dragged off to become a medic in the army. When the war was over he returned only to find that the college where he had hoped to study had been disbanded. He took up employment as an industrial chemist in a cement works.

One day at the factory a man fell from a height and was badly injured. While they waited for the ambulance Tom laid his hands on the man and applied a few of the moves he had been practicing. The man instantly could feel that his pain had lessened. The trauma had gone from his body. Others who watched were fascinated. As time went by Tom was asked more and more to practice his hands on therapy. His reputation as a healer grew. By the early fifties he had given up the job at the cement works and opened his own clinic. In essence he was a practising therapist without any formal training. Quite how he perfected this 'gift' is a bit of a mystery. However, I have my own theory.

Geelong has, or at least did have, quite a large Chinese population. As we are well aware the Chinese were ahead of us in medical terms years ago. Today we are just beginning to understand the benefits of acupuncture, yet it has been used in China for around three thousand, five hundred years. (General medicine in the United Kingdom officially accepted acupuncture in 1977). Of course once the medical profession had the authority from their superiors they embraced the modality with gusto. The consequence is that today many doctors, as well as being qualified GPs are qualified acupuncturists. Western medicine is now working hard trying to catch up with medical practices perfected in China eons ago.

But to my theory about Tom: An example of Chinese medicine that I remember from childhood was when I would spend happy hours watching American cowboy and Indian movies. The story would be that a gunman in battle had been injured with an arrow that had penetrated his shoulder. For whatever reason it seemed (in every movie) the practice was to break off the flight from the arrow but to leave the arrow head lodged in the flesh. Thus one of his fellow cowboys having removed the shaft and the flight from the arrow would sit and comfort the wounded man while another cowboy would run off to collect the Chinese man from the local laundry.

Copious amounts of whisky would be administered to the injured man, in an effort to take at least some of the pain from the on-site surgery that was about to be enacted. Removing the barbed arrowhead, still bedded deep in the tissue would I imagine be a painful exercise.The Chinese man would arrive, puffing and panting. Clad in traditional white suite, complete with a little round white hat perched on the top of his head and respite with a long entwined slender ponytail that would hang from the nape of his neck it would often be seen to curl all the way down to his waist. This form of dress was typical of what we were led to believe was the distinctive dress for someone from the East at that time of life.

The Chinese man (or part-time surgeon) would then take out a knife. He would put the blade into a flame to sterilise it and burn off any bacteria. Allowing that the whisky had had little effect as an anaesthetic the cowboy would howl as the Chinese man would cut open the flesh around the wound. Apparently the arrows used by the Red Indians (as I knew them to be) were nasty things in that they had a barb on the end, which meant that if you tore it from the flesh it would cause all sorts of damage to muscle and connective tissue. Nonetheless as a lad, seated in a little old cinema in Ardrossan, staring a big screen, I could see that whatever the Chinese man was doing was painful. The shriek from the cowboy simply reinforced my opinion.

Even in my youth the Chinese were accepted as being a wise nation. Thus this little sensible Chinese man knew that the wound had to be cauterised to prevent bacteria from entering. Basically he had to seal the flesh and provide a barrier from the atmosphere. He had to make it sterile. So, he would bite a bullet in two and sprinkle the contents, the gunpowder, over the open wound. Striking a match he would flash it at the wound. The gunpowder would explode and in the process scorch the flesh. Thus it would be cauterised.

In the West we were slow on the uptake of this important form of medicine. The days of Florence Nightingale working trying to help the unfortunates who had been wounded in the Crimean War are not that far back. During that time, people died after amputation and other brutal bits of surgery that were administered. The wounds would suppurate and infection would enter simply because they had not been cauterised. There was no barrier to stop bacteria.

The Chinese invented gunpowder a long time ago. Yet how on earth did the Chinese man know that he had to burn the flesh around the wound to help the body to heal? Who taught him?

Was it a case that this and other bits of medicine had been handed down through the ages? The fact is that in today's hospitals open wounds are cauterised after surgery. The doctors don't use gunpowder. They use an electrical device, which is heated and has a hot tip. The skin is burned to seal it and coagulates bleeding points too small to be closed with ligatures (a thread for tying round a vessel for restricting the flow of blood).

As a result it is my opinion that what we are doing today with medicine in the West is simply what the Chinese developed all those thousands of years ago. My theory is that Tom may well have spoken with his Chinese friends in Geelong; befriended them. In the process he might have learned the basics of the therapy he developed. He could well have been sifting the brains of some old Chinese sage. Much as I have, he may have had a brain that continually asks who, how, where, why, what and when. Today we accept that some of the most potent drugs in the world are derived from ancient Chinese medicine. As I write these words I understand that a number of laboratories in different parts of the world are underway with experiments to prove the efficacy of such old-fashioned treatments. Tom I suppose in his own way was the catalyst for a (Chinese) health-care revolution.

By 1974 the success of what he had developed had spread far and wide in Australia. It seems that Tom Bowen never advertised the merits of the work that he did at his clinic, yet by then he was treating around 13,000 patients per year in his one-man clinic. Considering that treatments were usually 7 days apart and that most people needed two or three visits, that was an amazing number of patients per year. It has of course to be accepted that Tom had 5 treatment rooms and with the help of some nurses that worked with him, treated five patients at a time. Accordingly he came under investigation by the Australian federal government. They placed two of their medical researchers in his clinic to examine what he did.

They stayed with him for six months. At the end of the study, they came to the conclusion that he was doing nothing wrong. Thus today, in Australia, New Zealand and other parts of the world you will find a Bowen therapist in almost every town. Around the world we now have in excess of 10,000 therapists.

Tom taught only a few therapists. In 1974 he met one of them, Oswald Rentsch (Ossie), a natural therapist practising massage and osteopathy. Over the next two years Ossie became one of Tom's apprentices and scribe, documenting his treatment protocols. Ossie then started using Bowen's technique in the town of Hamilton, Victoria, where he and his wife operated their own clinic. It was not until after Bowen's death in 1982 that he started to practice and eventually teach what would come to be known as the Bowen Technique.

How then does Bowen work you may ask?

Bowen is described as an original system of powerful soft tissue mobilisations that affect the body both structurally and energetically to restore its self-healing mechanism. We all have this ability, but sometimes the body forgets. Your traffic lights are on red. Energy simply will not get to where it is needed.

A Bowen therapist will put the traffic lights back onto green, restoring the body's ability to heal. The body understands Bowen as a language that it knows and accepts that we are resetting the body to heal it.

It is painless, non invasive and safe to use on anyone from newborns to the elderly. It provides long lasting relief from a wide range of acute and chronic conditions. Bowen moves are made with the fingers with simple rolling moves over the skin and fascia of muscles, ligaments or tendons on various but precise parts of the body. Fascia is under the skin and is what wraps us up. It encloses every muscle ligament and tendon inside us and keeps the various soft tissue parts of our bodies separate from one another.

In an effort to explain fascia I would ask you to think of an orange. Peel off the outer skin. What you then see are segments of flesh separated from one another by a thin membrane. This thin membrane is much like the fascia that wraps up all of our muscles. Unlike the membrane surrounding the individual orange segments it is very strong. Surgeons will use it to stitch us together, internally, after they have operated. In all there is a bewildering array of different layers, yet the arrangement is simple in design.

It is true to say that some of the Bowen moves are made over acupuncture points: some actually cross over two or three at a time. Perhaps this may help explain my theory about Tom studying with the Chinese and their use of acupuncture often placed on the meridian lines on the body. More to the point is that fact that Bowen works on the autonomic nervous system and is probably where the body's self-healing mechanisms are governed. The autonomic system controls over 80% of the bodies functions and is very susceptible to external stressors. It controls all of the involuntary actions. How you salivate, how you blink, how you digest your food, how your heart beats and so on. You don't have much, if any, control over this. Let me give you an example:

If I were to cut out your heart, put it in a bath of warm blood and feed it with some glucose it would continue to beat at a regular pace for quite a long time. The heart has this ability. However, when you run, the body needs an increased supply of blood, oxygen and nutrients. The heart has a need to speed up. A part of the brain at the back of the head (the medulla) is connected by way of a nerve loop system to a point at the top of the heart called the sino-atrial (SA) node. This node is located in the wall of the right atrium. It is a small region of specialised tissue, which exhibits spontaneous excitation. In a way it is the hearts pacemaker and initiates electrical impulses which make heart muscle cells contract at a certain rate.

So, if you are climbing a flight of stairs, the medulla sends a message down a nerve to the SA node which in turn tells the heart to speed up. The converse of this is that at night when you go to bed and you don't need the heart pumping so quickly, another message comes down the same route and tells the heart to slow down. These signals are passed in the autonomic nervous system.

The point is though that we don't have much, if any, control over this, yet this is the system that Bowen uses to send a message from the muscle or ligament or tendon, which is being energised.

Bowen stimulates the proprio receptive responses in muscles tendons and some joints. It works on the natural feed back loops within the muscles and tendons by actuating the muscle spindles and the golgi tendons via the spinal tracts to various parts of the brain, including the cerebellum, the thalamus, the putamen (the area concerned with co-ordination of muscles) and the brain stem. However, let us not get too complicated in all of this terminology. Simply stated the therapy works. Of course at this point I am happy to state that after a career change and completion of my studies both here and in Australia I have my own clinic in Glasgow. (Address, and contact details at the end of the book).

Of course my story is far from finished. My studies and work with Napier University are in their infancy, but indeed BNT is my Holy Grail. The perfect end to my little tale! In this story I hope that I have explained how I came to terms with my back pain affliction. How I searched for a 'cure', how I allowed myself to be used and abused by so-called back pain experts and indeed when my future at one stage offered nothing other than life in a wheelchair, I was certainly in the depths of despair. In all of this I strived for my 'Holy Grail'. I knew that it was out there somewhere. I never gave up. Finding Bowen therapy was a miracle in itself. A one in a million chance!

Bowen has totally changed my life. It has made me whole again. I can enjoy my times on the golf course without fear of my back muscles going into spasm. Now that I am older and wiser I never venture onto the first tee without my warm up exercise. Often at my golf club when performing my warm-up routine in the locker room my fellow golfers look at me with quizzical looks. Perhaps they think that I am silly. Yet, on the first tee I am the one who knocks a pain free drive twenty yards further than my partners.

Life in all has become an enjoyment again. I look forward to each and every day accepting that God will have the final say in how many he gives me. I have great joy in spreading the gospel of Bowen Neural Therapy to the people in Scotland or indeed anyone who will listen to me. It gives me enormous pleasure to work in my clinic making people whole again. The fact that I can make people better and resolve their health problems is wonderful. Using BNT as a tool is the best thing that has ever happened to me. I cannot speak too highly of the modality. The excellent thing is that it works. The additional fact that we may soon have clinical trials to prove the efficacy will give the therapy credence. In time all doctors indeed hopefully the whole of the medical profession will accept the worth of BNT, not just the five doctors and two Glasgow surgeons that I currently have as patients.

I had occasion recently to converse by e-mail with Ossie. He wrote me these words: "The fact will always remain that Bowtech the Original Bowen Technique understood and used correctly is all that you need". With this I can only concur.

Of course I continue to have regular treatments myself. My philosophy is that we all have our cars serviced regularly. Why then don't we have our bodies serviced in the same manner, or is it simply a case that we only look for a treatment when we are ill?

Patients come to my clinic in Glasgow for treatment. Initially they have a problem, which I will try to resolve. I am not able to help everyone; to be sure I would be a fool if I suggested that I could do so. The documented success rate in Bowen treatments is written as somewhere around an 84% success. Pretty high!

Most folk who come to my clinic will experience relief from their problem. Once we have reached this status I then ask the patient to move on to some form of maintenance agreement. Some patients agree to come once or twice a year much as we will do when we have our teeth cleaned at the hygienist. Others attend once every couple of months. Some of my MS patients come every two weeks to keep their systems in condition.

BNT in other words is preventative. Some of my patients find the therapy to be so rewarding that they have been attending the clinic on a regular basis for years. Thus, like I do, they accept that prevention is better than cure. Since I had my first treatment I can honestly state that my back muscles have since never once gone into spasm. To me this is worth more than a million dollars. Better than winning the lottery! What can any one of us do if we don't have health? Without it a man or a woman has nothing.

From what I read in the press, life expectancy is increasing by two years every decade. The Ancient Roman man counted himself lucky if he lived to 23, while modern day man can expect to live to 75. Of course as I have written in an earlier chapter, the rich will have access to life-prolonging therapies while the poor will still die young. Yet in all of us life is preferable to death, but achieving long life has its own health issues that we will have to deal with. Of course there is research into stem-cell treatment and such, but this science is as yet unproved. Spare part surgery is a fact of life as is the therapy that I practice. It seems that much of the damage that accumulates through life tends to blossom in later life. Sadly, this applies particularly to those of us that suffer with back pain. This makes it all the more important to have regular therapy treatments so that our later years are healthy and well spent.

There is though one other man who deserves a mention. Gene Dobkin lives in San Jacinto, California, USA. He was one of the original Bowen instructors and seemingly having the same inquisitive mind as I have he spent time in Australia studying not just with Ossie but also speaking with and asking every bit of explanation available from the five others that studied with Tom. I laugh when I think of the story that Gene told me about the problem we have with the fragmentation of Bowen and the fact that too many 'leaders' insist that theirs is the original form. Thus it was that he found himself in Geelong reverently standing at the graveside staring at the ground and wondering what he could have asked Tom were he still alive. However, as he stood he smiled at the thought that he would dig him up.

Then at his next class he would be able to hold up the remains and proclaim that indeed he did have the real Tom Bowen!

Gene wrote two manuals about Bowen that I have found fascinating. Truly excellent in-depth analysis of his teachings, I would urge anyone who has an interest in the subject to purchase a copy. (See Bibliography: A Bowen Home Companion). Thus, it was that I became an admirer of Gene Dobkin. To me it seemed that he was able to give answers that the Academy wouldn't or just downright refused to give. Here in the marvellous volumes written by Gene, were the answers to many of the questions that my Bowen instructors were unable to give.

As a result, inspired, I invited Gene to come to the UK in August 2005 to teach and to give me and others willing to learn from him the benefits of the therapy that he has developed known as Neural Touch. He has returned since in August 2006 and is due to visit these shores again in March 2007.

He teaches the meaning of universal laws: The law of Assumption: The Law of Similars: The Law of Polarity: The Law of Unity: The Law of Reversed Effort: The Law of Duplication. All of which I knew little, yet all of which have so much to do with the ongoing chemical factory that is inside every human being. Like reading the line of a put on a green, the eye will instantly give the correct route, yet within not many seconds later the brain will try to convince you of another; a complexity in the multifaceted world of the human being that few of us are able to comprehend, or understand.

To say that Gene is a genius is perhaps overstating matters. However, much like Tom, he is intuitive and gifted. What I like about his teaching is that he tells his students to think about what he has developed and indeed challenges them to see if they can improve on his technique. Gene is pushing the medical barriers ahead with all sorts of imaginative ideas. To quote from Gene's Bowen Bridge manual: "It is wished that the student take these techniques not merely as a set of directives, but also as a springboard to customize your sessions. This is the living legacy that Tom Bowen left us, and which we would be well advised to continue. Any piece of any technique may be extracted and used as a spot treatment of its own or placed in another context within a session. Make the technique your own."

The therapy that I now practice is a blend of not just the original Bowen taught by Ossie but also what I have learned from Gene and indeed other developments that I have made myself. In this my thanks go equally to Gene and to Ossie. Together with my research that will commence shortly, in collaboration with Napier University, Edinburgh, and the blossoming of the Bowen Neural Therapy Society (a group of like-minded therapists committed to research) I look to the future with relish. I accept the wisdom that the original Bowen must be taught in a 'pure' fashion as it was left to us by Tom Bowen. This though doesn't prevent us from pushing the barriers ahead in research. Thankfully I have a brain that will continue to ask who, how, where, why, what and when of everything that touches me, much like the Glasgow surgeon who has recently perfected keyhole surgery for heart by-pass. This procedure once involved opening the chest cavity with all the risk and trauma that surrounded it, but he has now developed a technique that allows just a tiny hole to be cut and microscopic instruments and camera to be inserted into the heart to affect the repair. The patient is allowed home the next day rather than having to spend days, or weeks even, in intensive care.

I am deeply grateful for the training that I received from the Bowen Therapy Academy of Australia and humbly accept the gift that they passed from Tom Bowen to me. I do hope that they won't be angry at my desire to push the barriers just that little bit further. My reason for this is to prove the efficacy of BNT and more importantly in doing so to convince the Scottish Executive and the Health Service here in Scotland that the use of this therapy can save them money rather than having doctors prescribe yet more pills, the cost of which is prohibitive. More importantly, the integration of this therapy into the NHS will allow everyone in Scotland (and other countries that will follow their lead) to appreciate the benefits of a therapy that only the fortunate few who can afford to pay are allowed to enjoy. Then, truly I will have reached my goal in life and will perhaps be likened to Tom Bowen who was seen as an osteopathic grandfather who was pleased to help the poor and to do so without charge.

I have a mountain of bureaucracy to get through to achieve this and a lot of hard work in the process. But with the help of God, Sheila and other good folk who are willing to work with me I am sure that together we can achieve the impossible.

So as they say in Disney World 'That's all Folks!' The end of my story but I hope the beginning of the end of your own back pain.

Take on board the advice I have given in this book and get down to your local practitioner as soon as you can or give me a call at my clinic where I will be delighted to help with your problem and discuss your own concerns. No matter where you are in the world there will be a therapist somewhere near you. The worst bit of your life is now behind you. The best is yet to come.

If there is anything in this book that you don't understand, or anyone that I have introduced without proper explanation, I will be pleased to respond to your comments, and give answers, such that you will fully understand the words written.

James Steele BTAA MGCP
The Bowen Neural Therapy Clinic
Glasgow
Scotland

www.bnth.org where you will find the information that will allow you to contact me.

I will be happy to answer any of your questions.

Other useful web sites:

www.usbowen.com (Gene Dobkin)
www.bowtech.com (Oswald Rentsch)
www.bowentherapists.com
www.complimentaryalternatives.com
www.garynull.com

Bibliography

House of Lords, Select Committee on Science
and Technology
Session 1999-2000 6th Report
Complimentary and Alternative Medicine
London – The Stationery Office

Managing Injuries in Professional Football
The roles of the club doctor and
physiotherapist
Centre for Research into Sport and Society,
University of Leicester, 1999.

Janet G Travell MD and David G Simons MD
Myofascial Pain and Dysfunction
Lippincot Williams and Wilkins, 1993

Frederic H Martini
Fundamentals of Anatomy and Physiology,
Seventh Edition
Pearson, Benjamin, Cummings, 2006

Andrew Beil LMP
Trail Guide to the Body
Andrew Biel, 1997

Donald W Novey MD
Clinicians Complete Reference to
Complementary and Alternative Medicine
Mosby Inc, 2000

Noel M Tidy
Massage and Remedial Exercises
Simpkin Marshall, 1944

Gene Dobkin
A Bowen Home Companion
Omniquest Inc, 1998

Neil A Campbell
Biology Fourth Edition,
Benjamins Cummings Publishing Inc, 1996

Michael Murray MD and Joseph Pizzorno ND
Encyclopaedia of Natural Medicine
Little Brown, 2002

Gordon Waddell
The Back Pain Revolution
Churchill Livingstone 1998

Michel Guérard
Cuisine Minceur
Éditions Robert Laffont S.A. Paris 1976